Library and Information *Sources and Services*

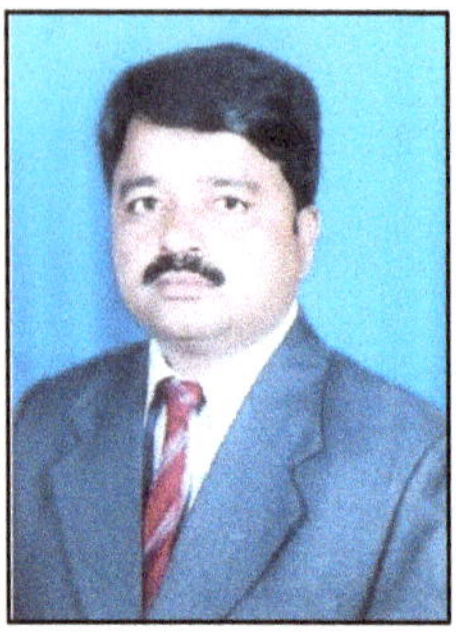

Dr. U.S. Jadhav, Assistant Librarian, Karnataka Veterinary, Animal and Fisheries Sciences University, Bidar have put up 15 years of library experience. He has published several articles in National and International books. He was awarded Gold Medal in M.Phil from Gulbarga University; Gulbarga and he obtained Ph.D. in 2010 from Gulbarga University, Gulbarga. Also he is life member of National Library Associations like Indian Library Association, Indian Association of Special Library and Information Centre and SALIS and Association of Agricultural Librarians and Documentalists of India (AALDI).

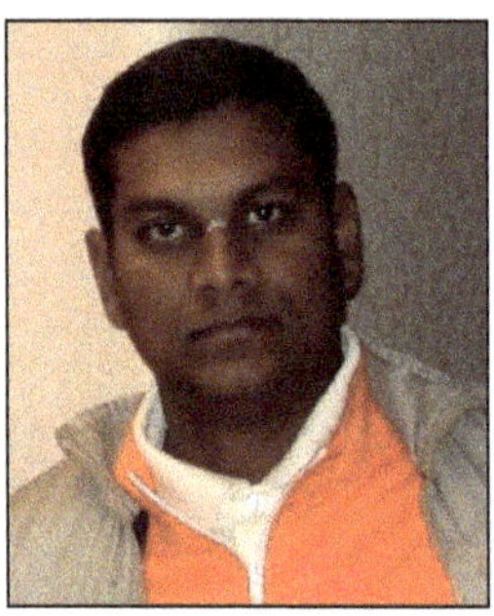

Dr. Suresh Jange, Deputy Librarian, presently working in Virtual Learning Resource Centre and Digital Library of Gulbarga University, Karnataka, has fifteen years of professional experience. He was awarded Gold Medals in B.L.I.Sc and M.L.I.Sc, and passed the UGC NET exam. He served earlier at ETDC (Dept of Electronics), Hyderabad, and Tata Institute of Social Sciences, Mumbai.

Jange has published 80 research papers in Indian and foreign journals, festschrift volumes, and presented papers at national and international conferences. He received IFLA-ALP fellowship in 2007 and visited Victoria University, Wellington, New Zealand. He also visited and presented papers at Nanyang Technological University, Singapore (2006), and Karolinska University, Stockholm, Sweden (2005).

Library and Information
Sources and Services

– Authors –

U.S. Jadhav

Assistant Librarian,

Karnataka Veterinary, Animal and Fisheries Sciences University

Bidar, Karnataka

Suresh Jange

Deputy Librarian

Virtual Learning Resource Centre and

Digital Library of Gulbarga University,

Karnataka

2012

REGENCY PUBLICATIONS

New Delhi - 110 002

ISBN 9789351240914

Published by : **REGENCY PUBLICATIONS**
(*Division of Daya Publishing House*)
4760-61/23, Ansari Road, Darya Ganj,
New Delhi - 110 002
Phone: 23245578, 23244987
Fax: (011) 23260116
e-mail : info@regency-books.com
website : www.dayabooks.com
website : www.regencybooks.com

Laser Typesetting : **Classic Computer Services**
Delhi - 110 035

Printed at : **Chawla Offset Printers**
Delhi - 110 052

PRINTED IN INDIA

Karnataka Veterinary, Animal & Fisheries Sciences University
P. B. No. 6, Nandinagar, Bidar - 585 401, Karnataka

Prof. Suresh S. Honnappagol
Ph.D., FISSAR, FNAVSc, FISACP, FIAAVR
Vice Chancellor

Ph: 08482 245264
Fax : 08482 245107
e-mail: vckvafsu@yahoo.co.in
sskvafsu@yahoo.co.in
www.kvafsu.edu.in

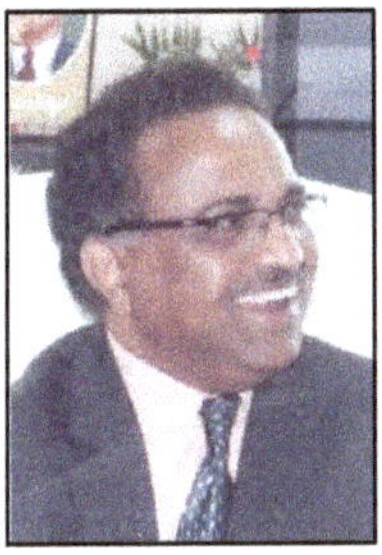

Ref. No. *VC/USJ/2011-12/II-2609* ***Date*** *01-07-2011*

Foreword

I am very happy to go through the book, *"Library and Information Sources and Services"* By *Dr. U.S. Jadhav,* Assistant Librarian, Karnataka Veterinary, Animal and Fisheries Sciences University, Bidar and *Dr. Suresh Jange,* Deputy Librarian, Gulbarga University, Gulbarga. This book would be of immense value and useful for library science professionals including agricultural sciences, policy makers and IT professionals to explore the various information sources including internet technology, e-resources and databases in meeting the timely information needs of the society. This book is also of high value to the agricultural and veterinary scientists to meet the syllabus of Library and Information services recommended by ICAR, New Delhi [compulsory non-credit course *PGS-501 Library and Information Services (0+1)*] and it is helpful to students/scientists/faculty members to equip the library users with skills to identify, collect, formulate search and use various information sources including Internet, OPAC, CD-ROM and online, databases.

Dr. V.S. Jadhav and Dr. Suresh Jange have taken keen interest in writing this book on library services, which is very useful to equip the library users to trace information from libraries efficiently, to apprise them of information and knowledge resources, to carry out literature survey, to formulate information search strategies, and to use modern tools of information.

(Suresh S. Honnappagol)
Vice Chancellor
Vice-Chancellor
Karnataka Veterinary,
Animal and Fisheries Sciences
University, BIDAR

Preface

Higher education is witnessing transition from to learner; faculty centered to learner centered institutions; teaching to the design and management of learning experiences; and from student to a lifelong member of a learning community and all these suggests changes in teaching and learning process. For this, Library and Information science play a pivotal role in enhancing quality education, research and development. In the present ever increasing growth of scientific literature, emerging research fronts, interdisciplinary, extra disciplinary research programs and publications of varied types of learning resources, networks, and logical creative and critical approaches in the curriculum, the academic libraries constitute as an integral part of education system in catering to the diversified information needs of the society with its rich information sources and services.

Libraries have always been considered as the channels of information centers. The value of the library is found in its collection of information resources. Earlier, the libraries were acquiring information in paper and print form, so that it could be disseminated to the clientele. As the volume of information is growing and the traditional means of transmitting information is changing, libraries are expending their traditional roles to survive and flourish in an electronic age. Today, more emphasis is being given on the electronic format of information for obvious reasons. The Internet has emerged as a *de facto* global distribution medium for electronic information sources. Web publications from university campus sites and pre-print archives are flourishing on the Net. Refereed journal, articles and article abstracts are increasingly accessible via web delivery from commercial publishers, research libraries and other intermediaries. Most of the abstracting databases accessible in CD/ DVD format are made available online as well. Subject guides for the higher education and research community, providing links to high quality Internet resources, are becoming increasingly important discovery tools. It is packed with both primary and secondary sources of information, to track, which one has to develop the ability to sift through millions of search engines hits. Most of the information products – data, reports and research papers and national consortia resources are increasingly created in digital form distributed universally through the various Net services.

Mere possessing variety of information sources that includes primary, secondary and tertiary sources both print and electronic media is of hardly any use, unless systematic Library and information services are extended to the users for optimum utilization of resources in the library. In fact, Library services have changed dramatically from traditional mode of services to techno-based services with the advent of sophisticated technologies in the millennium. Developing search skills are important in identifying and retrieving right information at the right time. Information skills today include, but also go beyond, the traditional skills needed to select a topic, conduct scholarly research, and compose one's ideas and map to the information sources. To achieve this, suitable search strategies depending upon the type of information and sources have to be adopted. Further, technological innovation has lead to provide services like online reservation of books, self issue/ return, virtual reference service, user instruction, document delivery, access to consortia e-resources remotely etc. The present book would be of immense value library science professionals, policy makers, computer science and management professionals to understand different types of information sources including Internet technology, e-resources and databases; concept of library, information services, literature search and citation manuals, Internet and online sources, organization and retrieval tools for making efficient use of library sources and services. To meet the syllabus of Library and Information services recommended by ICAR, New Delhi to equip the library users with skills to identify, collect, formulate search and use various information sources including e-resources on the internet, this book is of great value to the agricultural and veterinary scientists pursuing their studies.

Dr. U.S. Jadhav

Dr. Suresh Jange

Contents

Chapter 1
Library and Information Services

1.1 Evolution of Libraries

Libraries form a vital part of the world's system of education and information storage and retrieval. These libraries make available the information through books, manuscripts, journals, films, recordings and other media the knowledge that has been accumulated through the ages. People in all walks of life use library resources in their work for education, research, teaching, planning and development. Libraries are the temple of knowledge plays a very important role since the ages in the development of civilization, betterment of humankind and march of science. It is very difficult to trace the origin of library, but a lot is known about some of the most celebrated libraries in the ancient world.

The history of libraries begins concurrently to the history of the written record, as human beings developed methods of recording information on cave walls, stone, tree bar, or other media; the accumulation of written records, including clay tablets, papyrus rolls, parchment, and paper, provoked a need for convenient storage, access, and preservation. In fact the history of libraries can be traced back to the ancient era when our forefathers learnt the art of communication and writing, penned the information, knowledge and wisdom in the form of texts and manuscripts which carried the legacy of traditions, customs and knowledge from one generation to another. The earliest knowledge hubs of Nalanda, Taxila learning centers spread the fragrance of knowledge, enticed the knowledge seekers across the terrestrial boundaries. Library at Ninevah, the capital of Assyria founded in 7th century BC contained thousands of clay tablets and the famous Library at Alexandria in Egypt created by Ptolemy Soter during 3rd century BC contained the major part of the world's recorded knowledge in papyrus rolls.

In the evolution of human civilization, Agricultural Revolution, Industrial Revolution and Information revolution have played a very important role. Alvin Toffler, Peter Drucker, Regis Debray, and others agree that the new information age is in the process of rapidly replacing the industrial era. This new phase of information and new technologies, the science and knowledge are becoming the critical factors of the so-called "value added" economy. That's how Alvin Toffler in his famous book "Third Wave" rightly observed that the computer and communication technologies are leading us to the "Third Wave," a change of information age, electronic era creating the concept of global village.

Library's primary role is to provide access to books, journals and other sources of information including non-print sources. Access to information is the prime concern rather than preservation. The traditional methods now have been integrated at the electronic frontier to facilitate rapid transfer of information on a global scale. Advances in computer storage and telecommunication methods, online access to databases, electronic journals, electronic knowledge banks, document delivery, teletext, teleconferences, bulletin boards, CDROMS, networks etc., have been the revolutionary advances in the last two decades, that have brought a great change in communication, storing and handling of information. Thus, the library and information centers are the preservers of knowledge for posterity and use to support the information requirements of the society.

1.2 Concept of Library

The word 'Library' is derived the Latin word, 'Libraria', which means a place where books and other writings are kept. But the library of today is much more than a building stocked with books. Libraries are the treasure house with an open door. It is a workshop for the user community to accumulate knowledge and wisdom to step into a world of adventure in pursuance of academic and research endeavor.

According to Dr. S. R. Ranganathan, the father of Library Science in India, Libraries are not more store houses, they are rich springs from which knowledge flows out to irrigate the wide field of education and culture.

UNESCO's terminology of Documentation, Library is an organized collection of printed books and periodicals or of any other graphic or audio-visual materials and the service of a staff to provide and facilitate the use of such materials as are required to meet the informational, research, educational or recreational needs of its users.

Library does not mean merely a collection of books, but it is a learned institution equipped with treasures of knowledge maintained, organized, and managed by trained personnel to educate the children, men and women continuously and assist in their self-improvement. The Library is a trinity of documents both print and electronic, users/ readers/ scientists and library staff. Libraries from time immemorial have changed in their nomenclature from chained libraries to storehouse of information is called as Documentation centers, Information centers, Information clearinghouses, Information brokers, Gatekeepers, Knowledge centers, Learning Resource centers etc.

Due to the impact of Information Technology, the libraries are now moving towards "Learning Resource Centers". The modern libraries, the intellectual focal point in a sense are the digital and hybrid libraries and knowledge preservation and dissemination have rapidly changed especially due to the impact of technological revolution. Unlike simply providing access to books and journals, the modern libraries acquire digital tapes, CDROM databases, electronic books, and software to handle numerical data, audio, video and provide access to web pages, e-journals, FTP sites, Bulletin Boards, Internet etc. Thus the mission of the libraries is to:

- Develop information/knowledge resources focused on patron's needs.
- Organize information resources in-print and non-print considering the changing needs.
- Develop a co-operative user centered culture.

- Provide human and technologically moderate access to information.
- Provide continuing education and training to its users.

A useful way to explore the essence of libraries is to examine how users view "Goodness" in the library context. What is that makes a good library? formalized by Orr (1973) suggested two questions need to be asked "How Good is this Library" and "How much Good does this Library do". Today this could be more likely labelled as to effectiveness, efficiency, economy and impact questions. The question of goodness can also be related to adoptability and responsiveness of libraries to its environment.

Thus Library performance could broadly be ascertained through:

- **Integration:** Level of integration between mission aims and objectives of the institutions and those of library.
- **User satisfactions:** Document delivery, information services, study facilities and information skills program.
- **Delivery and Access:** Service standards development targets, skill development programs and mechanism to provide access to information timely.
- **Efficiency:** Outputs related to resources input.
- **Economy:** Cost per unit.

Also the timelines, relevance, aesthetics, reliability and other factors add to the effectiveness of a good library. Organization of sources, information delivery, training in information skill, customer-client-patron relations, works of imagination, creative ideas and services, best practices, etc. are other factors that increase the effectiveness of a good library.

1.3 Laws of Library Science

The development of any discipline depends upon the major contributions of individuals from time to time to bring to the limelight of other disciplines on par with excellence. In the field of Librarianship, Dr S.R. Ranganathan's contributions are quite innovative and ever remembered for the prosperity and visibility of library profession. In fact, today the libraries have reached a stage, which is considered as an integral part of any institution, is just because of a great visionary Dr S.R. Ranganathan. His five laws of library science in 1928 and published in 1931 are the first fundamental laws in the field of library science. Ranganathan's five laws essentially constitute a fundamental contribution to the development of Library Science which are relevant in the past, present and future developments.

These laws contain a philosophy of librarianship that harmonizes with the concept of service to increase the utility of graphic records for the benefit of the society. Thus the five laws of library science are found to be useful in providing logical interpretation of the present and future library practices and services. The five laws are:

- Books are for use
- Every reader his/her book
- Every book its reader
- Save the time of the reader
- Library is a growing organism

Books are for Use

In the past, the books were often chained to prevent their removal and that the emphasis was on storage and preservation rather than use. Without the use of materials, there is little value in the item. By emphasizing use, Ranganathan refocused the attention of the field to access-related issues, such as the library's location, loan policies, hours and days of operation, as well as such modalities as library furniture and the quality of staffing. This law seems to be very simple statement, but is self evident and advocates to the concept of an open stack library and furnishing useful books is the library. This law dictates the development of systems that accommodate the use of library materials.

Every Reader his or her Book

The second law emphasizes on the users of a library as prime importance. This law preaches that "Books are for all" and broadens the concept that books are not merely for few users but for all including poor, sick, blind, prisoner, neo literates and old irrespective of caste, creed and religion. Every member of the user community should be able to obtain materials as and when needed. Ranganathan felt that all individuals from all social environments were entitled to library service, and that the basis of library use was education, to which all were entitled. Librarians should have excellent first-hand knowledge of the people to be served. Collections should meet the special interests of the community, and libraries should promote and advertise their services extensively to attract a wide range of users.

Every Book its Reader

This principle is closely related to the second law but it focuses on the Books itself. This law desires that every book in a library must find its reader. It implies that there should be maximum use of books by their users. Appropriate arrangement of materials in open stacks also is an important means of achieving this objective of the third law. This law has implications on book selection, shelf arrangement, cataloging, reference service, accessibility, open access and extension service. Ranganathan argued that the library could devise many methods to ensure that each item finds its appropriate reader user of the library.

Save the Time of the Reader

Time is money and this fourth law recognizes the essence of extending quality services to the users of library to meet their academic and research needs. To this end, Ranganathan recommended the use of appropriate methods to improve library management. The collection must be arranged in an inviting, clear, and obvious way so as to save the time of patrons/ readers as they search for the materials they need. Well-planned and executed library handbooks, stack guides, automation and library tours, or research instruction sessions serve the goal of saving the time of the reader. Adequate staffing of reference, information, and circulation desks, as well as telephone reference, also helps patrons find needed materials quickly.

The Library is a Growing Organism

A library will grow in terms of documents, readers and staff. Dr Ranganathan argued that library organizations must accommodate growth in staff, the physical collection, and patron use. This involved allowing for growth in the physical building, reading areas, shelving, and in space for the catalogue. This law has implications on extension of library building, storage and weeding, choice of a classification scheme, shelf arrangement, and physical form of a catalogue, choice of a catalog code, reference service, user education, library orientation, and staff.

In the present changing information industry, M. Gorman's laws are the most famous in which he reinterpreted Ranganathan's laws in the context of today's library and its likely future providing his five new laws of librarianship:

- *Libraries serve humanity.*
- *Respect all forms by which knowledge is communicated.*
- *Use technology intelligently to enhance service.*
- *Protect free access to knowledge; and*
- *Honor the past and create the future.*

1.4 Types of Libraries

The Libraries are categorized into five types *viz*:

1. Academic Library
2. Public Library
3. Special Library
4. National Library
5. Contact Library

1.4.1 Academic Libraries

Academic Libraries comprise of school libraries, college libraries, and university libraries whose prime objective is to meet the academic needs of the particular institution for which it is created to serve.

School Libraries are meant for children's of young age of about 5-12 years of age and the teachers who are involved in teaching and shaping them. The school library should aim to foster book mindedness, strengthen learning skills through kits now available in plenty, create a love for books and other learning resources and inculcate the habit of reading.

College Library aims to meet the information needs of college students may be Pre-university College or Degree College lays foundation of a good and more responsible life in the future to support class room teaching. The libraries will therefore become equally important than the classrooms. These libraries will become students' workshops plays a very responsible role in satisfying the academic needs of young students.

The purpose of a **University Library** differs, in varying degree, from that of a school or college library in that the former adheres extensive and particular emphasis to research projects apart from the curricular needs of the institution. The University Library is a knowledge Centre for accessibility provides user focused services to obtain and evaluate scholarly information and knowledge available in main formats and strives to create new knowledge to increase understanding and develop wisdom to the students, research scholars and teaching faculty at post graduate and research level. The University Library provides access to specialized information resources and services to meet the academic and research information needs of the reading community by developing specialized need based collection; organizing information resources; providing access to human and technologically moderated access and orienting users to locate, obtain and evaluate information. The university libraries have a big responsibility and a very important role to play in shaping students for higher learning and research.

1.4.2 Public Library

This is often called a "peoples' university", a democratic institution operated for the people by the people that conserves and organizes human knowledge in order to place it freely in the service of the community without any distinction of occupation, creed, class, or race. It is a university of the people since it is maintained and financed by the people of the community who freely throng in this institution and acquire knowledge that they need in their day-to-day life. The scope of a public library meets general requirements of the public thus remains quite broader in its vision. It differs from the other types of libraries by offering opportunities of informal self-education and inculcates reading habit amongst all types of general readers and, as a consequence, maintains a sizeable collection of light literatures, i.e., fictions, novels, story books, etc., for recreational studies, and a children's corner.

1.4.3 Special Library

Special Library by the name itself indicate specialized in a particular field of knowledge differs in its mandate from other types of libraries on the grounds of collection of information sources, the type of users and services offered. It is concerned with literature of a particular subject or group of subjects, an institution which is 'created to serve the needs of some working organization, a company, a research association or a government department'. *e.g.* Library and Information Service Division, Bhabha Atomic Research Centre, Mumbai.

1.4.4 National Libraries

These are countries apex body preserving all the documents published in India for posterity and use. As per the Delivery of Books and Newspapers (Public Libraries) Act, 1954, National Library at Kolkata and its branch libraries in India are entitled to receive a copy of every publication brought out by anyone anywhere in the country. It is the apex body of the library system of India serving as a public library, it is a permanent repository of all documents published in India.

1.4.5 Contact Libraries

These are the libraries of other countries established in other parts of the world which aims at promoting a better understanding of the policies, values, institutions, and culture of their respective country by its collections. For instance, The American Library having four centers at Delhi, Chennai, Kolkata and Mumbai established in India provides with a wide range of current, accurate and authoritative information from a vast selection of print and electronic resources using state-of-the-art technology. Also, British Council Library, India focuses on learning and teaching English, Education, Library and information services, Arts and culture, Rights and society and Science.

1.5 Role of Libraries in Education and Research

Education, research and extension are the mandatory areas of activity of the university. Research and development contributions are to be extended to the beneficiaries through various government departments – Agriculture, Animal Husbandry and Dairy Development - various boards, corporations and other institutions. The scientists of the future must be armed with new knowledge, which will be different from that needed today. They will need more knowledge in the emerging disciplines of agriculture, veterinary science and public health. Free movement of persons and services are amongst the major democratic principles of any profession. Education and library are two inseparable indivisible concepts, both being fundamentally and synchronically related to and co-existent with each other. One cannot be separated from the other, and the existence of one is impossible without the other. None of them is an end in itself; rather both of them together are a means to an ultimate end. This inter-relation, this co-existence, this dependence of one upon the other have been coming down from the birth of human civilization to the posterity through a process of evolution in accordance with varied needs, changes, and circumstances of various stages of human life. The libraries are primarily responsible for the provision of academic information to support learning, teaching, research and extension.

Education aims to impart knowledge while libraries support education system serving as the repositories of knowledge providing access to timely needs of the users. Libraries have a long history, starting with the chained and closed-access libraries of earlier times to the present day hybrid, digital, and virtual libraries that use the latest technology for provision of information through various services. Accordingly, librarians have also changed from storekeepers who were concerned with protection of books against theft, mutilation, and pilferage, to that of information officers, navigators, and cybrarians who find themselves in the vast ocean of reading material and are busy in satisfying information needs of their clients.

With the advent of information and communication technology, the nature of libraries has changed dramatically. Computers are being used in libraries to process, store, retrieve and disseminate information. As a result, the traditional concept of library is being redefined from a place to access books to one which houses the most advanced media including CD-ROM, Internet, and provides remote access to a wide range of resources. Libraries have now metamorphosed into digital institutions. Gone are the days when a library was judged by its quantitative resources. Today, libraries are surrounded by networked data connected to vast ocean of Internet-based information sources and services.

The traditionally custodial role of the librarian is changing and use of technological innovations for cataloguing, information retrieval, and housekeeping procedures is commonplace, and the emphasis is increasingly on electronic resources especially with the development of national consortia like UGC Infonet, INDEST or CeRA. Never before have there been so many opportunities for involvement in an information-based society including electronic and multimedia publishing; local, national, and global networking; development of navigational and filtering tools for access to networked and non-electronic sources.

1.5.1 Technologists: From Practice to Informed Practice

The knowledge that "new era librarians" bring to this knowledge environment would make sense of a multiplicity of digital collections and resources, provide access to a network of key contacts, identify cost-effective strategies for information retrieval, and assist users in the publication and creation of new knowledge. Several personal characteristics plus the new skills and competencies are essential for the new era librarians to create and manage library collections and services. Demonstrated skills and sophisticated expertise competencies are needed for new era librarians to manage the Digital Information System (DIS) in the important areas of imaging technologies, optical character recognition, markup languages, cataloguing, multimedia indexing, database technology, user interface design, programming, and Web technologies.

It is ironical that all these technologies are under way, but not yet fully coordinated and targeted at the task of creating a new era librarian or digital librarian. The new era librarian will become the guardian of digital information and will be the vehicle to preserve democratic access to information. The librarian's role will be increasingly towards offering consultancy to the users in their efforts in providing digital reference services, electronic information services, navigating, searching and retrieval of digitized information through Web documents that span the Universal Digital Library or the Global Digital Library. The new era librarian will be an embodiment of a digital information professional or digital knowledge worker, who will ensure that the digital libraries are used effectively and with ease. Digital librarians with newly acquired skills can play a meaningful and leading role in the networked information society of the millennium. New era librarians add values and can make libraries truly useful and user friendly.

Nevertheless, printed materials will remain important and places to hold them will be necessary. It is hoped we can stay focus in this fast changing environment which demands that librarians and information professionals must be someone with multi-skills, multi-tasking abilities, and competent in areas of work such as management, communication, language, public relations and others. With the advent of virtual technologies, some librarians might see themselves as facilitators, matching up users in need of information with experts in a given field:

- ✰ ***Technology and tradition:*** Information and research resources are becoming more varied, most obviously as electronic products–materials converted from analog to digital formats and also materials that were "born digital"– become ever more pervasive.
- ✰ ***Technology and profits:*** Information resources, including those available electronically as well as many printed journals are more and more regarded as commodities rather than public goods.
- ✰ ***Technology and law:*** New means to deliver information, most particularly over the Internet, combined with the commodification of information resources, have undermined longstanding understandings concerning scholarly and educational access to research resources.

1.5.2 Media Specialist: From Actions to Evidence

Traditionally librarian is known as a person located in the library building carrying out the tasks like acquiring, organizing, preserving the printed documents besides helping the readers in locating the information needed by them. In the last decades of the twentieth century this picture has rapidly changed under the influence of advances in computer and communication fields. The paper collections have given place to networked, computer resident, user searchable collections like bibliographic databases, Online Public Access Catalogues (OPAC) obliterating the need for the user to visit the library building. With the digitization of ever increasing number of collections and advances made in computer/ communication hardware and software seamless access to digitized information located in geographically diverse locations has become a reality. The walls of library are thus pulled down and a "Virtual Library" in Cyber Space came into being. The Virtual Library brought in its wake new flavors in the form of digitizing not only printed material but also pictures, maps, scenarios, paintings and sounds and presenting them all in a lively show in a theatre like environment. Where do librarians stand in this scenario and where their profession is headed is the nagging question faced by one and all in the profession.

The use of new media is not only a technological issue. New media mean new ways of communication. As an example the choice of online synchronous 'chat services' in libraries implies an accelerated and more speedy way of communication. There is no time for the thorough interview or the careful information retrieval. The discourse of conversation in Instant Messaging (IM) is not straight professional. Especially conversations with young users may have a personal, cheerful or even private turn.

1.5.3 Researcher: Renewable Leadership

New era librarians are knowledge-based practitioners who use research as a foundation for their own professional practice and who support the conduct of research through their professional associations. Research has shown that the provision of appropriate information can lead to: better informed decision-making; the ability to proceed to the next step in a project or task; improved relations with a client; and the exploitation of new business opportunities. The right information at the right time can also benefit the organization by saving the time of highly paid employees, avoiding poor business decisions, and even direct loss of funds.

The rapid acquisition of so many new web-based resources was exhilarating and even enviable but it did pose serious problems. Adapting to such a large number of new resources within the course of a single academic year was a potential source of confusion and stress, not just to the research community but also to Library staff, who were expected to learn how to use the resources competently; to write help-sheets for users; to incorporate the new resources into user education programs; and to provide user support – in short, to become the instant "experts". It was extremely important that academic librarians were kept informed of developments and were involved in all decisions about which new resources were acquired.

It was equally crucial that they had a say in the matter and retained a degree of control. As there were a few initial expressions of concern about the unreliability of the web and about both the suitability and the stability of electronic resources, it was evident that another key responsibility of the librarian should be communication – not just with researchers but also with Library staff.

Keeping Library staff informed of developments has proved fairly straightforward. There were already many established channels of communication, ranging from regular formal meetings to an electronic in-house discussion list, lib-matters. Any announcements of new resources, changes to existing resources and other news can be posted to lib-matters and immediately reach each and every member of Library staff. In addition, regular visits to each site library to talk with Library staff about local needs and problems as well as research activities helped to overcome the barrier imposed by working at some distance from one another.

Informing researchers of developments proved more problematic. Librarians agreed to highlight the new services in their user education programs, meetings, and informal encounters with research staff and students. Even so the librarian felt the need to develop a method of reaching researchers directly, systematically and regularly. The library can provide the e-mail addresses of the research coordinators. But e-mailing these individuals each time when there was a new development in their discipline proved haphazard and ineffective. Following discussion with researchers, a more methodical method of communication was identified one intended not only to communicate announcements of new services but also to educate researchers about Library services in general and to stimulate a two-way flow of information.

Thus, academic librarians proficient and knowledgeable in the identification, location and evaluation of information, have an even greater role to guide faculty, students and other users in the best use of both print and online resources in the library. This can have a significant impact on student learning: making them aware of the potential for useless and inferior information available on the Web; recognising the distinction between information from refereed scholarly journals, grey literature, unrefereed digital information, misinformation and disinformation; and resisting total reliance upon convenient information from the Internet.

India is essentially an agrarian society and basically depends on agricultural outputs. It is therefore essentially that the technology thrust should lay greater emphasis on the transfer of scientific and technological information from the research institutes to its actual users. Libraries and Information Centres are playing a very important role in providing information to the users by building print and electronic collection. Indian Council of Agricultural Education and Veterinary Council of India are the two important national bodies striving to achieve excellence in higher education and developing national educational policies in India.

Libraries of Agriculture and Veterinary institutions have been providing academic support to its scientists by ensuring quality based library and information service and assisting in the academic, research and extension activities of the institutions. However, numerous problems are faced by these libraries in the Indian context, *viz.*, financial crunch, lack of adequate infrastructure, technological gadgets, manpower, technical competencies, escalating cost of the literature, ever changing needs of the users, devaluation of Indian currency in the international market etc. Moreover, electronic resources relevant to the profession are developing at an unprecedented pace. Academic libraries are considered to be the nerve centers of academic institutions, must support teaching, research, and other academic programmes.

The establishment of the Indian Council of Agricultural Education (ICAE) under the Indian Council of Agricultural Research (ICAR) was one of the major steps undertaken by the Government of India. It helped the development of Agricultural education including animal science education in post- independence period. The decision to set up the council was taken in a conference of state ministers of Agriculture convened by the ICAR in November 1951 as per the recommendations made by the Agricultural Education Committee of the Central Advisory Board of Education which felt with the growth of a large and comprehensive system of agricultural education, it has become necessary that the institutions concerned maintained proper standards of instruction and training.

With the independence of India, various teams reviewed agriculture education and research. The Agriculture Review Committee, which consisted of eminent scientists from India, the United Kingdom, and the United States, recommended the reorganization of agricultural and veterinary education in India. Based on their report, a series of agriculture universities were established beginning in 1960. The Uttar Pradesh Agricultural University was the first of these, established at Pantnagar in 1960; other states followed. In certain states implementation was either slow or half-hearted, and the universities did not always get the full support of their state governments. This stunted the growth of these universities, leading to inadequate progress in the field of veterinary education and research. Financial support to these universities by the state governments was reduced, and budget allotted by the authorities to veterinary and fisheries faculties was, and remains both meager and disproportionate to the gross national product contributed by these sectors. The deterioration of veterinary and fisheries education under an agricultural universities set-up led to the establishment of separate universities for veterinary and animal sciences, including fisheries, at Tamil Nadu in Chennai in 1989, at Calcutta in west Bengal in 1995, at Nagpur in Maharashtra in 2001, at Bidar, in Karnataka in 2004, in the Andhra Pradesh states at Tirupati in 2005; and most recently in Punjab state at Ludhiana in 2006. More veterinary universities are in the offering in the near future in many other states.

The Veterinary Council of India is a statutory body of the Government of India framed under an Act of Parliament *i.e.* Indian Veterinary Council Act, 1984 (52 of 1984). This is an Act to regulate Veterinary practice and Veterinary education. The Act stands extended to all the States of India. Only those who possess recognized veterinary qualification and registered can practice in the country. Since its inception the VCI has been taking active steps in revising the curriculum in collaboration with the ICAR and its adoption by the universities. This council advises the Central and State Government on all the matters related to veterinary education and practice.

Today there are forty three veterinary colleges under different universities spread all over India and are under the control of Veterinary Council of India act which was formed during year 1989 with the concept of uniform syllabus with minimum standards in all the states. They are conceived to act as leaders in veterinary education to train the manpower and promote the veterinary education in the country. However, with the advancement of veterinary science and establishment of Veterinary Council of India, it was strongly felt to give autonomous status to this science through establishment of separate Veterinary and Animal Science University. Thus, at present there are one university under the ICAR system *i.e.* Indian Veterinary Research Institute (IVRI), Izatnagar while at state level there are six full fledged Veterinary and Animal science Universities namely, Tamil Nadu Veterinary and Animal Science University, Chennai established in the year 1989, West Bengal University of Animal and Fisheries Sciences, Kolkatta established in 1995, Maharashtra State Veterinary University established in the year 2000 at Nagpur, Karnataka Veterinary, Animal and Fisheries Sciences University, Bidar established in the year 2005, Sri Venkateshwara University of Veterinary and Animal Sciences at Tirupati in 2006 and very recently Guru Angad Dev Veterinary, Animal and Fisheries Sciences University in 2007 at Ludhiana. It is expected that such independent veterinary universities will also come up in every state to promote veterinary and animal sciences.

1.6 Library Services

The success of any library system depends upon the effectiveness and efficiency of information services rendered to the scientists to meet their educational and research endeavor. The information service that provides the assistance to the users by libraries using information technology automatically search on most recent entries in a database for the benefit of users is termed as info-tech based information services. As such libraries attached to the institutions of higher learning like Agriculture, veterinary and other research institutes should extend the information services as under:

1.6.1 Circulation Service (Issue/Return/Reserve)

Circulation is a prime service of issue/ return books on fixed period of time to the scientists for home taking purpose. This service also makes provision for reserving the book facility which has been lent out to users.

1.6.2 Reference Service

Reference services are the personal assistance offered to the scientists (users) to help them to define and identify correctly, bearing in mind how he/she intends to use the information. Reference tools like dictionaries, encyclopaedias, directories, indexes, abstracts etc.

readily available in the library or information unit, may be used for rendering reference services.

1.6.3 Referral Service

Referral services are the directing services or the guiding services about the availability of information sources. These services do not provide the scientists with the information sources or documents needed but refer him or her to the sources such as secondary publications, information units, professional organizations, research institutes and individual specialists, library etc.

1.6.4 Current Awareness Service (CAS)

In order to keep the scientists abreast of latest developments in their respective field of research that has recently been published and added to the libraries, the library head needs to inform the scientists for utilization of new collections in the library. To accomplish this purpose, information products at various intervals of time are issued in the form of bulletins like Current Additions or Content alert services or displaying new arrivals on the shelf. This service will keep the scientists well informed about the new collections in the library and enable in promoting the use of library sources and services. Selective dissemination of information is a refined method of supplying each user or a group of users with the references of documents or abstracts relating to their predefined areas of interest matching the users profile and new documents published recently and received in the library.

1.6.5 Textbook - Reserve Shelf

Textbooks are purely subject oriented books which are recommended by the subject experts and are issued to the scientists in addition to the general collections of the library. Normally the number of textbooks issued to the user is restricted to one or two unlike general reading books.

1.6.6 SC/ST Book Bank

With a motto to help the students belonging to Scheduled Caste and Scheduled Tribes, a separate unit is being provisioned in almost all the academic libraries known as SC/ST Book Bank, wherein books are lent out to these students for a semester/ academic year in addition to the general book collections.

1.6.7 Literature Search

Literature search service is considered as an extension of reference service and is undertaken by the library staff on behalf of the user scientists that includes compilation of bibliographies, searching CD-ROM databases and online databases. Much of the expertise in literature searching depends on identification and choosing the most appropriate sources to be searched and the order of searching them. Expertise in literature search can be developed only by experience. Knowledge of the subject field of search would be an asset in providing literature search service. On-line databases and CD-ROMs are increasingly being used for providing literature searches.

1.6.8 Web-OPAC

The library is a service-oriented institution which facilitates the users with its rich information resources through catalogue. The development of information technology and library software's in different platforms has enabled the library and information centers to host their bibliographical records on the Internet termed as Web OPAC. The OPAC in the networked environment is confined to the users within a campus, whereas the Web-OPAC extends its identity to the world by making its resources made available in the bibliographical format. Now the library holdings are not only confined to library premises, but it hosted on the Internet revealing the collections of the library to the world. This facilitates the users to search the availability of documents in the library irrespective of location either by author, title, subject, etc.

1.6.9 Internet Services

Internet is now considered as online library due to its wealth of information sources and services available on the Internet. The information sources includes e-books, e-journals, e-newspapers, e-reference sources, e-patents and other online databases including national consortia based information products. Today Internet service has become integral part of library services to the scientists. The Internet allows us to share information and resources such as, government documents, electronic journals, electronic books, media publishing, human anatomical images, computer software, bibliographic and full-text databases, speeches, live concerts, audio and video clippings.

1.6.10 Access to Consortia Electronic Resources

The primary purpose of establishing a library consortium is to share physical resources including books and periodicals amongst members. However, the mode of cooperation has gone under a transformation with infusion of new information technology from print-based environment to digital environment known as consortia. In this context, various national consortia's have been established mainly to overcome financial crunch and to share the e-journals, e-books and e-databases at a nominal charges among group of libraries. Some of the national consortiums available in India are UGC Infonet, CeRa, INDEST consortia etc.

1.6.11 Indexing and Abstracting Services (CD-ROMs/Online Databases)

Due to the development of information technology, information is increasingly recorded in digital format and electronic databases which are continually becoming more complex, information storage and retrieval as the technology obsolete very fast, CD-ROM is also facing problems due to emergence of the DVD. In today's business, education, and government environments the amount of information, data and software being archived and distributed on CD-ROM and DVD-ROM media is overwhelming. Most of indexing, abstracting and full text databases are now available in CD/DVD format like BIOSIS, VET-CD, AGRIS (The International Information System for the Agricultural Science and Technology Database) etc.

1.6.12 Document Delivery Service (DDS)

Document Delivery Service is an improved version over Inter-Library loan in the networked environment. To fulfill the information needs of the end user through information/document supply is a document delivery service. Under this service, the copies of papers from learned journals, conference proceedings and other materials available in their collection at nominal cost or free are made available to the scientists on request. Documentary delivery systems are to be developed at Indian Agricultural Research Institute (IARI), National Dairy Research Institute (NDRI), Indian Veterinary Research Institute (IVRI), Central Institute of Fisheries education (CIFE) and State Agricultural Universities (SAU's) to enable those Consortium partners who do not have the print versions of particular scientific articles. Information and Library Network (INLIBNET) has initiated interlibrary loans and document delivery services from the comprehensive collection of subscribed journals under JCCC@UGC-INFONET. This sort of document delivery services is also available for INDEST consortia and CeRA consortia.

1.6.13 Reprography Services

Reprography refers to Xeroxing of library information sources is provided on nominal charges to the user/scientists. Reprography service is the most common service rendered to the Faculty, Students and staff only.

1.6.14 User Education and Sensitization Programmes

Academic libraries support the teaching and research needs of institutions they serve. It is the libraries' responsibility to ensure that the use of its information sources, resources and services are optimized to benefit its users, hence the necessity for libraries to conduct user education and sensitization programmes as a regular feature. This will facilitate optimum utilization of existing library resources facilities and services.

References and Further Readings

Brophy P. and Coulling, K. (1996). Quality management for information and library managers. London: Gower.

Brophy, Peter. (2000). The Academic Library, London: CA, 224 P.

Brophy, Peter. (2001). Library in the 21st Century: New Services for the information age. London: Library Association, 201 P.

Gaddagimath, R.B. (1997-98). Information Management Skills for Users in Indian Agricultural Libraries: An in depth study on resources, curriculum design and development of learner's packages. Ph.D. Thesis, Karnataka University.

Gorman, G.E. (Ed.) (2000,). International Yearbook of Library and Information Management 2000-2001: Collection Management, London: Library Association, 464 P.

Gorman M. (1998). The five laws of library science: then and now. School Library Journal, 44(7): Jul, p20-23.

Hardison, O. B. *Jr.* (1989). Disappearing through the skylight: Culture and technology in the twentieth century: Viking Penguin.

Harle, (2009). Jonathan Dazzling technologies: the libraries place. ACU Bulletin 167, 30-31.

National Assessment and Accreditation Council, Bangalore, India, Library and Information Services: Case presentations. Best practice Series No. 2, 2006, Pp80.

Orr, R. H. (1973). Measuring the goodness of library services: A general framework for considering quantitative measures. *Journal of Documentation*, 29 (3), 315-332.

Quality Assurance Agency for Higher Education, UK. Librarianship and information management: Subject Benchmark Statements. http:// www.qaa.ac.uk/benchmark/library.pdf.

Ranganathan S R. (1988). Five laws of library science/2nd edn. Bangalore: SRELS,

Ranganathan, S.R. (1931). The Five Laws of Library Science: Madras Library Association.

Roberts, S.A. (2001). Trends and developments in financial management of collections in academic and research libraries: The Bottom Line: *Managing Library Finances*, 14(3),152-164.

SCONUL. Information skills in higher education. SCONUL position paper. (www.sconul.ac.uk/publications/99104Rev1.doc).

Veterinary Council of India. Available at www.vci.nic.in (Accessed on 14th May, 2011).

Chapter 2

Information Sources

2.1 Introduction

Information is sine-qua-non for the development and prosperity of a society. Information plays a significant role in all aspects of human activity whether it is education, research and development, business and industry, government affairs. Today, a country is considered prosperous, in socio-economic terms, if it is rich in information especially in the field of science and technology that's why the concept of information rich country and information poor country are categorized. Information has become a basic resource, and as such, information generated should be procured, organized, and disseminated properly to support to the varied needs of the society.

Historically, communication in science was achieved through one-to-one communication. During 1455, the invention of movable printing by Gutenberg in Germany brought a revolution in the history of written communication has led to the production and dissemination of multiple copies of manuscripts. Today, the ongoing information explosion has created a situation where it's now impossible for any one person to stay up-to-date with the changes in any subject contributing to existing body of knowledge resulting information explosion.

2.2 Types Sources

Information is a life blood of modern research and essential tool for academic and research community. In order to obtain useful information on any assignment or topic, one need to identify what kind of information is required and right kind of information sources. Information sources are the sources from where information is derived to meet various needs. Information sources are available in different types and they are categorized into three type's *i.e.*

- Primary sources
- Secondary sources
- Tertiary sources

The different types of information sources available under: primary, secondary and tertiary sources are depicted below.

Primary Sources	*Secondary Sources*	*Tertiary Sources*
Periodicals	Textbooks	Directories
Research Reports	Dictionaries	Yearbooks
Trade Literature	Encyclopaedias	Bibliography of Bibliographies
Thesis/ Dissertations	Indexing and Abstracting Sources	
Conference Proceedings	Handbooks/ Manuals	
Patents		
Standards		

2.2.1 Primary Sources

Primary sources are primary in nature and the results of original invention being produced in different forms of primary sources. These primary sources are the first published records of original research and development activities and represent the original unfiltered ideas and comprise of the most recent available information.

Periodicals

The most popular medium of publishing results of research and developmental activities is through periodicals. Thus periodicals form the bulk of primary source literature of science and technology. Periodicals include journals, bulletins, transactions, proceedings, and other serial publications, which appear regularly. The contents of periodicals vary in the kind of material included and in technical level as well.

Periodicals by the name itself indicate that any written information that comes out periodically that includes Newspapers, Magazines, and Journals are all periodicals. The articles within periodicals tend to be more specific or about certain aspects of an issue in comparison to the comprehensive nature of monographs.

Periodicals take many forms, including:

Newspapers usually offer articles that are factual accounts of events, but they can be an analysis of trends or issues as well. Newspaper articles usually are not written by experts in the field and do not offer suggested readings or reference the author's sources of information.

Magazines are the least scholarly type of periodicals, though in some cases consulting a popular magazine might be useful for tracking a current issue or trend or to assess social values and interests of a given population and time period.

Journals are scholarly or academic in nature and contain original research work published at a regular intervals and is also known as vehicle of scientific communication. Journal articles are written by researchers or academics and generally offer citations to the sources consulted. A peer-reviewed journal accepts manuscripts and sends them out to other experts in the field to evaluate the article.

Ex:

- ✰ *Behavioral Ecology*, Oxford University Press
- ✰ *Journal of Veterinary Behavior: Clinical Applications and Research*, Elsevier
- ✰ *Current Opinion in Clinical Nutrition and Metabolic Care*, Lippincott Williams and Wilkins (LWW)
- ✰ *Plant Journal*, Wiley-Blackwell Publishing

Research Reports

Research reports are the important primary source of information especially in science and technology. As compared to other primary sources, research reports are less polished form as they are produced early in the research process. These research reports are emerged as the most successful alternative sometimes to journals. Research reports are originated in research laboratories working under an organization pursuing research and development activities.

Ex:

- ☆ Research Report NIFS Technical Series. (1990). Japan: NIFS
- ☆ Research Reports on Information Sciences, Series A Mathematical Science. (2004). Tokyo: Institute of Technology.
- ☆ Research Report of Utilization of radiation by Isotope Users group. (2004). Japan: Japan Atomic Industrial Forum
- ☆ Research report of Utilization of radiation by medical users' group. (2004). Japan: Japan Atomic Industrial Forum.
- ☆ National Institute for fusion science. Research Report Tech series. (2004). Japan: National Institute for Fusion Science.

Patents

Patents are the significant form of primary source that contains results of original invention providing rights over the invention to the inventor. These patents are of immense valuable information source for invention, technology, business, and legal actions. More than one fourth of the technological and scientific publications produced every year are published by patent offices around the world. Modern researchers and technologists emphasize the need for rapid and accurate information; patent specifications meet such needs. Patents are used to evaluate specific technology, identify and alternate technology and its sources, improve an existing product or process, develop new products or processes, and monitor development in a specific technology. **E**uropean **P**atent **O**ffice (**EPO**) publishes **EPIDOS** (**E**uropean **P**atent **I**nformation and **Do**cument **S**ervice) database. It contains about over 33 millions references from 1968 onwards of all the patents filed and granted in approximately 71 countries. Almost 3 millions references are added each year. In India, offices of The Patent Information System (PIS) and National Institute of Intellectual Property Management (NIIPM) are at Nagpur looks after control of patents.

Ex:

- ☆ Crowne, J. D. (Ed.) (2000). *BNA's* Patent, Trademark and Copyright Journal.Washington: The Bureau of National Affairs.
- ☆ European Patents handbook. (2000). New York: Chartered Institute of Patent Agents.
- ☆ Food Patents Bulletin. (2000). England: Leatherhead Food R.A.
- ☆ Hughes on copyright and Industrial design. (2000). Canada: Butterworths.
- ☆ Patent office technical society Journal. (2000). Calcutta: Patent office technical Society.
- ☆ Saunderson, K. M. (1972). Patent as a source of technical information. Aslib Proceedings. 24, 244-254.

Standards and Specifications

Standards are one type of primary document that contains specifications or norms for quality, size, or shape of industrial products. These help in simplifying the product's distribution by a manufacturer and eliminating the non-standardized items from the market. These standards ensure quality of products and any product either consumer or other manufactured bearing standard mark like Indian Standard (IS) or British Standards ensures quality of the product. These standards and specifications plays significant role in centers like Standardization, Testing and Quality Certification (STQC) - INDIA

These are usually drawn up by organized agencies, governments, or quasi-governments like Bureau of Indian Standard (BIS) in India (http://www.bis.org.in/), British Standard Institute (BSI) in Britain, Bureau of Standards in USA etc. In India alone, BIS brings about 300 standards annually. Some of the standards in the field of science and technology are:

- ☆ Ramsey, C. G. (1998). Architectural graphic Standards for architects, engineers, decorators, builders and draftsmen. New York: John Wiley and Sons.
- ☆ British Standards Institution. (1955). Summaries of British Standards for building materials and components for housing. London: The Institution.

- ☆ Society of Motor manufacturers and traders. (1957). Standards for the British automobile industry. London: The Society.
- ☆ Maule, R.W. (1997). Information networks and services: an over view of foundations, Standards and practices for modern information management. California: Information Association Press.
- ☆ Kahin, B. and Abbate, J. (Eds.). (1995). Standards policy for information infrastructure. Cambridge: MIT Press.

Some of the standards in the field of library science are:

Resource Description Formats

- ☆ MARC 21 formats - Representation and communication of descriptive metadata about information items.
- ☆ MARCXML - MARC 21 data in an XML structure.
- ☆ MODS (Metadata Object Description Standard) - XML markup for selected metadata from existing MARC 21 records as well as original resource description.
- ☆ MADS (Metadata Authority Description Standard) - XML markup for selected authority data from MARC21 records as well as original authority data.
- ☆ EAD (Encoded Archival Description) - XML markup designed for encoding finding aids.
- ☆ VRA Core – The VRA Core is a data standard and XML schema for the description of works of visual culture as well as the images that document them.

Digital Library Standards

- ☆ METS (Metadata Encoding and Transmission Standard) - Structure for encoding descriptive, administrative, and structural metadata.
- ☆ MIX (NISO Metadata for Images in XML) - XML schema for encoding technical data elements required to manage digital image collections.
- ☆ PREMIS (Preservation Metadata) - A data dictionary and supporting XML schemas for core preservation metadata needed to support the long-term preservation of digital materials.

- ☆ TextMD (Technical Metadata for Text) - XML schema that details technical metadata for text-based digital objects.
- ☆ ISO/DIS 25577 - Information and documentation – MarcXchange.
- ☆ ISO 20775 - Schema for Holdings Information.
- ☆ ALTO - Technical Metadata for Optical Character Recognition.
- ☆ AudioMD and VideoMD - XML Schemas that detail technical metadata for audio- and video-based digital objects.

Information Resource Retrieval Protocols

- ☆ Z39.50 - Supports information retrieval among different information systems.
- ☆ SRU/SRW (Search and Retrieve URL/Web Service) - Web services for search and retrieval based on Z39.50 semantics.
- ☆ CQL (Contextual Query Language) - Formal, user-friendly query language for use between information retrieval systems.

Standard in Progress

- ☆ Extended Date/Time Format (EDTF).

ISO Language Codes

- ☆ ISO 639-2: *Codes for the representation of names of languages– Part 2: Alpha-3 code.*
- ☆ ISO 639-5: *Codes for the representation of names of languages– Part 5: Alpha-3 code for language families and groups.*

International Standard Serial Number (ISSN)

- ☆ **Metadata for Digital Content**: Developing institutional policies and standards at the Library of Congress.

Trade Literature

Trade literature is the products of Industrial and commercial companies that produce trade literature, which constitutes an important form of primary sources of scientific and technical literature. Trade literature aims to illustrate and describe equipment or goods relating to the manufacturers. They are issued by the manufacturers or dealers and are often very well produced. Trade literature may take the form of a technical bulletin, price list, data sheet, etc. India is also one of the largest producers of trade literature that includes sheets, folders, pamphlets, and bound volumes containing original data on new products and processes. The trade literature collection is internationally known as an extraordinary source for the history of American business, technology, marketing, consumption, and design. Trade literature includes printed or handwritten documents, usually illustrated, of items offered for sale, ranging in size from small pamphlets to oversized folios of several hundred pages. The Role of Trade Literature in Sci-Tech Libraries addresses the problems of handling sci-tech trade literature in a corporate technical library, a large public library, and a government library.

- Pharmaceutical Manufacturing Review. (1996). England: Argus Business Media.
- Injection molding. (1993). Denver, CO: Canon Communications.
- International Polymer Processing. (1986). Germany: Hanser Verlag.
- Aviator Hotline. (2004). USA: Heartland Aviation Group.
- Pea and Bean Progress. (2004). London: Processors and Growers Research Organization.

Theses and Dissertations

Theses and dissertations are the products of the researchers carrying out research work for the award of degree. Theses and dissertations are rich and unique source of information, often the only source for research work that does not find its way into various publication channels. Doctoral dissertations are manifestation of result of four to five years of intense work involving huge investment of resources, both mental and physical and infrastructure and other support from the universities. They provide evidence from original research and thus form an important category of documents for the researchers in the concerned field. These are normally unpublished thesis submitted to universities and research institutes. In India, Shodhganga@INFLIBNET Centre available at

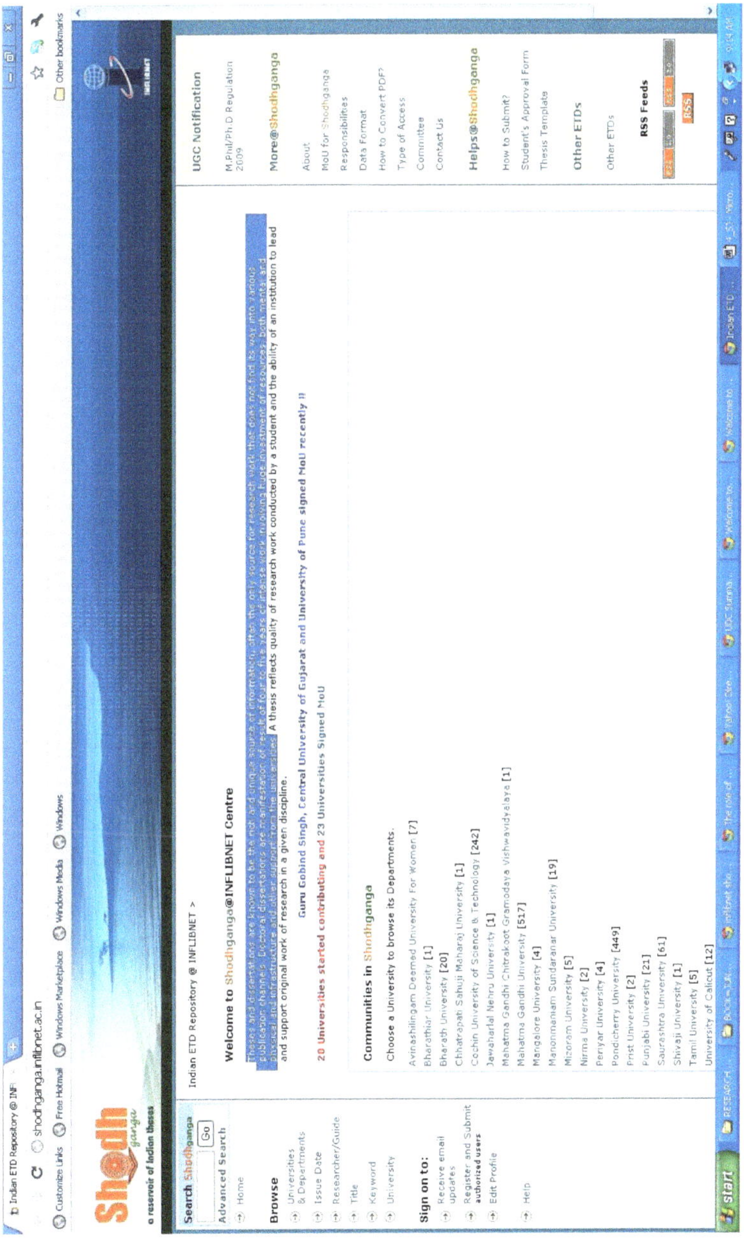
Indian ETD Repository @ INFLIBNET >
Welcome to Shodhganga@INFLIBNET Centre
Theses and dissertations are known to be the rich and unique source of information, often the only source for research work that does not find its way into various publication channels. Doctoral dissertations are manifestation of result of four to five years of intense work, involving huge investment of resources, both mental and physical and infrastructure and other support from the universities. A thesis reflects quality of research work conducted by a student and the ability of an institution to lead and support original work of research in a given discipline.
Guru Gobind Singh, Central University of Gujarat and University of Pune signed MoU recently !!
20 Universities started contributing and 23 Universities Signed MoU
Communities in Shodhganga
Choose a University to browse its Departments.
Avinashilingam Deemed University For Women [7]
Bharathiar University [1]
Bharath University [20]
Chhatrapati Sahuji Maharaj University [1]
Cochin University of Science & Technology [242]
Jawaharlal Nehru University [1]
Mahatma Gandhi Chitrakoot Gramodaya Vishwavidyalaya [1]
Mahatma Gandhi University [517]
Mangalore University [4]
Manonmaniam Sundaranar University [19]
Mizoram University [5]
Nirma University [2]
Periyar University [4]
Pondicherry University [449]
Prist University [2]
Punjabi University [21]
Saurashtra University [61]
Shivaji University [1]
Tamil University [5]
University of Calicut [12]
Shodhganga
a reservoir of Indian theses
Search Shodhganga
Go
Advanced Search
Home
Browse
Universities & Departments
Issue Date
Researcher/Guide
Title
Keyword
University
Sign on to:
Receive email updates
Register and Submit
authorized users
Edit Profile
Help
UGC Notification
M.Phil/Ph.D Regulation 2009
More@Shodhganga
About
MoU for Shodhganga
Responsibilities
Data Format
How to Convert PDF?
Type of Access
Committee
Contact Us
Helps@Shodhganga
How to Submit?
Student's Approval Form
Thesis Template
Other ETDs
Other ETDs
RSS Feeds
RSS

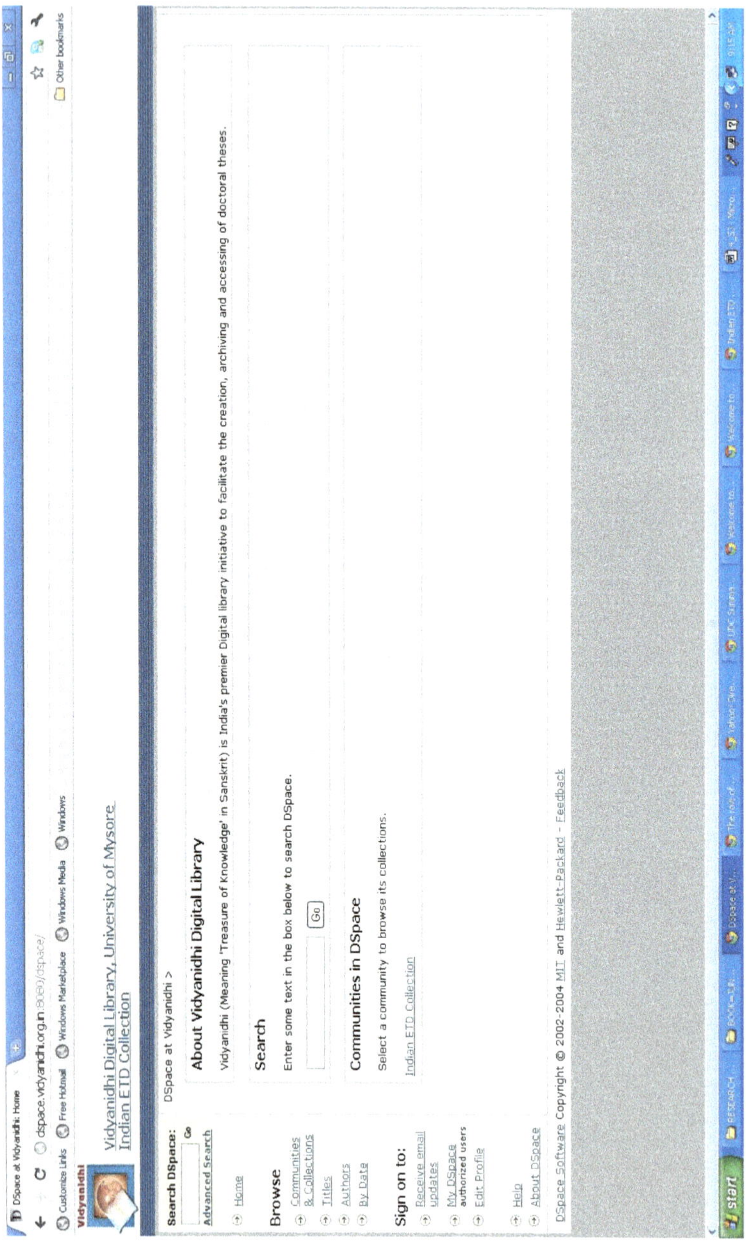
DSpace at Vidyanidhi: Home
dspace.vidyanidhi.org.in:8080/dspace/
Customize Links
Free Hotmail
Windows Marketplace
Windows Media
Windows
Other bookmarks
Vidyanidhi
Vidyanidhi Digital Library, University of Mysore
Indian ETD Collection
Search DSpace:
Go
Advanced Search
Home
Browse
Communities & Collections
Titles
Authors
By Date
Sign on to:
Receive email updates
My DSpace
authorized users
Edit Profile
Help
About DSpace
DSpace at Vidyanidhi >
About Vidyanidhi Digital Library
Vidyanidhi (Meaning 'Treasure of Knowledge' in Sanskrit) is India's premier Digital library initiative to facilitate the creation, archiving and accessing of doctoral theses.
Search
Enter some text in the box below to search DSpace.
Go
Communities in DSpace
Select a community to browse its collections.
Indian ETD Collection
DSpace Software Copyright © 2002-2004 MIT and Hewlett-Packard - Feedback
start

http://shodhganga.inflibnet.ac. in/) and Vidyanidhi (http://www.vidyanidhi.org.in/) envisioned to evolve as a national repository and a consortium for e-theses through participation and partnership with universities, academic institutions and other stake holders. Vidyanidhi enhances access to Indian theses and enlarges the reach and audience for Indian doctoral research works.

- ☆ Adams, M. L. (2003). Chemically tailored polymeric miscelles for drug delivery. Unpublished Ph.D. thesis, University of Wisconsin, Madison.
- ☆ Robertson, M. P. (2001). Engineered regulation of an RNA Ligase ribozyme. Unpublished Ph.D. thesis, University of Texas, Austin.
- ☆ Ackley, J. A. (1997). Weed management programs in potato, transported tomato and transplanted pepper with rimsulfuron and other herbicides. Unpublished Ph.D. thesis, Virginia Polytechnic Institute and State University, Virginia.
- ☆ Wang, Shensheng. (2001). Weighting normalization in optimal predictive control. Unpublished Ph.D. thesis, University of Missouri, Columbia.
- ☆ Bennett, Elena Michele. (2002). Patterns of Soil Phosphorus: concentrations and variability across an urbanizing agricultural landscape. Unpublished Ph.D. thesis, University of Wisconsin, Madison.

2.2.2 Secondary Sources

Due to increase in number of primary sources, a tool that helps to locate primary sources has led to the emergence of secondary sources. These are organized works and compilations that derive from or refer to primary source literature make up the secondary source of science and technology information. Secondary sources generally represent the "worked-over" knowledge rather than new knowledge and organize primary literature in a more convenient form. They not only serve as repositories of digested facts, but also act as bibliographical keys to the primary sources and sometimes these secondary sources replace primary sources as well.

Textbooks

Books are the intellectual work of an author which may be either textbook or general book either to suit general or subject oriented nature. Books are the monographic book typically provides with comprehensive information on a general topic, or at least more general information than what is found in an essay or article. A good monograph will give you a sense of the scope and historical background of an issue, as well as a thorough analysis of it. Textbook teaches the basic skills of open source development incrementally, through real involvement in meaningful projects, for students and self-learners. Textbooks analysis is the systematic analysis of the text materials including the structure, the focus, and special learning assists. Now a day, textbooks are available in electronic format known as e-books.

Ex:

- ☆ Ettinger, Stephen J. and Feldman, Edward C. (2010). Textbook of Veterinary Internal Medicine: Diseases of the Dog and Cat, 3rd Ed in 2 Volume. Philadelphia: Sounders, Pp- 2710

Encyclopaedias

An encyclopaedia is a type of reference work, a compendium holding a summary of information from either all branches of knowledge or a particular branch of knowledge. These are very useful source of information to the beginners to understand the background knowledge of any particular concept. Encyclopaedias are designed to give a summary of the background knowledge in a particular field which may be either general or subject based encyclopaedias. Scientists frequently turn to the encyclopaedia for their everyday information needs. They provide neither current nor exhaustive information, but furnish a vast wealth of facts which are easily found. Encyclopaedias act as a bridge between the world of scholars on one side and an individual in search of information on the other.

- ☆ Finn, F. and Robinson, E. K. (1999). International Encyclopaedia of Ornithology. Delhi: Biotech Books.
- ☆ Burton, M. and Burton, R. (1988). Encyclopaedia of the Animal Kingdom. London: Macdonald.
- ☆ Trivedi, P. C. (2000). Encyclopaedia Botanica. *Jaipur:* Pointer.

- *Cowles* Encyclopaedia of Science, Industry and technology. (1967). New York: Cowles Educational Corporation.
- Parker, S. P. (Ed.). (1982). McGraw-Hill Encyclopaedia of Chemistry (5th edn.). New York: McGraw-Hill Book Company.

Dictionaries

Dictionary is a collection of words of a language or a subject, arranged in alphabetical order with each word's meaning, spelling, pronunciation etc. In science and technology the purpose of a dictionary is to define commonly used terms in the simplest manner. Etymology and pronunciation of terms may be included too. Thesauri, dictionaries of synonyms, provide an effective language interface between the user and a storage system. They help by grouping words according to their meaning rather than alphabetically. Thesauri are different from dictionaries, as they do not contain meanings or definitions of words, except to a very limited extent in the form of scope notes and synonyms. Dictionaries can also be either general dictionary or subject based dictionaries.

- Singh, O. P., and Srivastava, S. K. (1998). Dictionary of Entomology Plant Pathology and Nematology. New Delhi: Concept Publishing.
- Sharma, R. (Ed.). (2003). Management terminology. New Delhi: Lakshay.
- Hartman-Peterson, P., and Pigford, J.N. (1991). Dictionary of Science. New Delhi: Universal Book Stall.
- Jain, A. (Ed.). (2003). Medical Terminology. New Delhi: Lakshay.
- Read, P. G. (1982). Dictionary of Gemology. London: Butterworth Scientific.

Indexing Services

An index is a systematic guide to the items contained in the book or journals or any source of information which may be either author index, title index or subject index. Index is also an alphabetical list of the names, terms, formulae, and other significant items in a completed work, along with page numbers where the particular terms are found and forms a backbone of any document.

The term 'indexed' is "derived from the stem of the Latin verb 'Decade' which means literally to show". The index serves two purposes: to minimize time and effort in finding information and to maximize the searching success of users. The index identifies the concepts or information present in a document and indicates their location in the volume. It gives users systematic and effective shortcuts to the information they need.

Ex: Science Citation Index

Science Citation Index provides researchers, administrators, faculty, and students with quick, powerful access to the bibliographic and citation information they need to find relevant, comprehensive research data. Overcome information overload and focus on essential data from over 3,700 of the world's leading scientific and technical journals across 100 disciplines. It is also available through *Web of Science®* and the online version, *SciSearch®* as *Science Citation Index Expanded®*, which covers more than 6,650 journals across 150 disciplines (http://thomsonreuters.com/). Science Citation Index helps to find high-impact articles from peer-reviewed and influential journals and keep up-to-date with the latest developments in one's respective field of research.

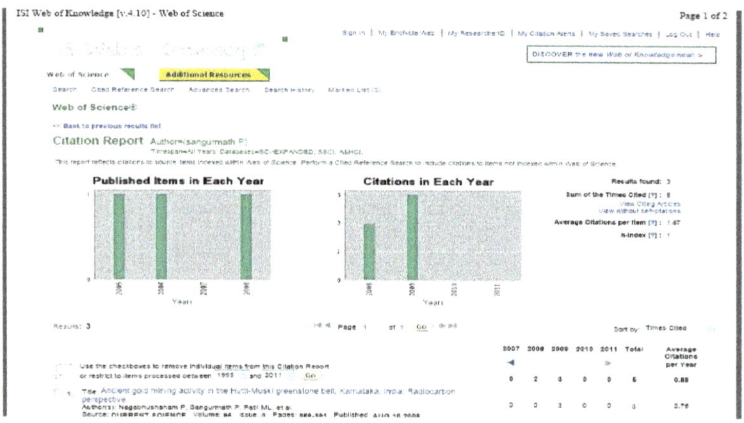

Abstracting Services

An abstract is a concise summary of original document. Abstracts are summaries of the content of publications or articles. Abstracting services act like a current awareness tool for the scientists or technologists, and perform a dual purpose by alerting them of newly published work, avoiding time consuming perusal of the original documents. They can act as surrogates when the original document is difficult to obtain. It helps the researcher save his time by grasping at the steadily rising tide of the publications.

Abstracts are of two types *i.e.* Indicative and Informative abstract. Indicative abstracts merely tell briefly what the document is about. It is a brief abstract or short summary written with the intension on enabling the reader to decide whether he/she should refer to the original publication or article Informative abstracts by name suggests that they are longer and present the essential data and conclusions so that the reader has no need to referee to the original document and sometimes substitute to original research paper. There are many abstracting sources or services are available in various subjects. Some of them are

Chemical Abstracts

CAS monitors, indexes, and abstracts the world's chemistry-related information, updating it daily and making it accessible through state-of-the-art information services. CAS databases offer many scientific disciplines, including biomedical sciences, chemistry, engineering, materials science and agricultural science. Chemical Abstracts is published since 1907 and is a weekly publication. It contains bibliographic information for approximately 80,000 publications. More than 155,000 entries, mainly for periodicals and facilitates searching by author name, keyword, CODEN, etc., for easy access to the bibliographic information

Biological Abstracts

Coverage: 1926 - Present

Broad and Specific Subjects:

- ☆ Life and Biomedical Sciences: Biochemistry and Biophysics; Biomedical Engineering; Biotechnology; Cell Biology; Development Biology; Microbiology; Molecular Biology.
- ☆ Pharmacology: Pharmacology.
- ☆ Science.
- ☆ Animal Sciences- Aquaculture and Fisheries, Zoology.

- ☆ Animal Sciences; Aquatic Sciences; Biodiversity Conservation; Biology.
- ☆ Earth and Geological Sciences- Agriculture, Botany, Ecology.
- ☆ Earth and Geological Sciences; Genetics and Genomics .

Online Equivalent:	Included in BIOSIS Previews
Print Equivalent:	Biological Abstracts
Data Type:	Bibliographic with Abstracts
Number of Records:	11.3 million
Records Added Annually:	250,000+
Interface:	OvidSP

CABI–Veterinary Science Database published by CABI

Coverage: 1973 - Present

Broad and Specific Subjects

- ☆ Arts and Humanities: Business and Economics
- ☆ Clinical Medicine: Nutrition and Dietetics
- ☆ Science:

  Animal Sciences- Veterinary Science;

  Animal Sciences;

  Earth and Geological Sciences- Plant Sciences, Forestry, Crop Science and Plant Biology, Crop Protection, Biotechnology, Plant Breeding and Genetic Resources, Agriculture;

  Earth and Geological Sciences; Genetics and Genomics

Print Equivalent:	Index Veterinarius; Veterinary Bulletin
Data Type:	Bibliographic with Abstracts
Number of Records:	650,000
Records Added Annually:	15,000
Interface:	OvidSP

The methods used for searching this database is shown in screenshots:

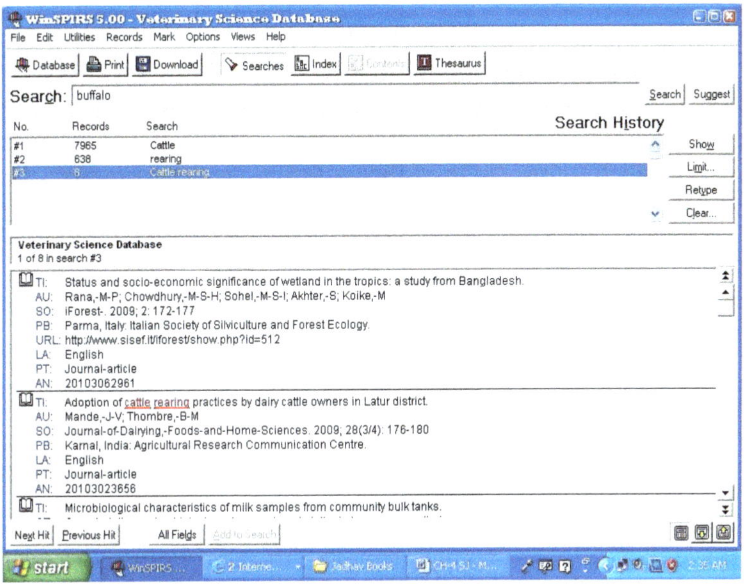

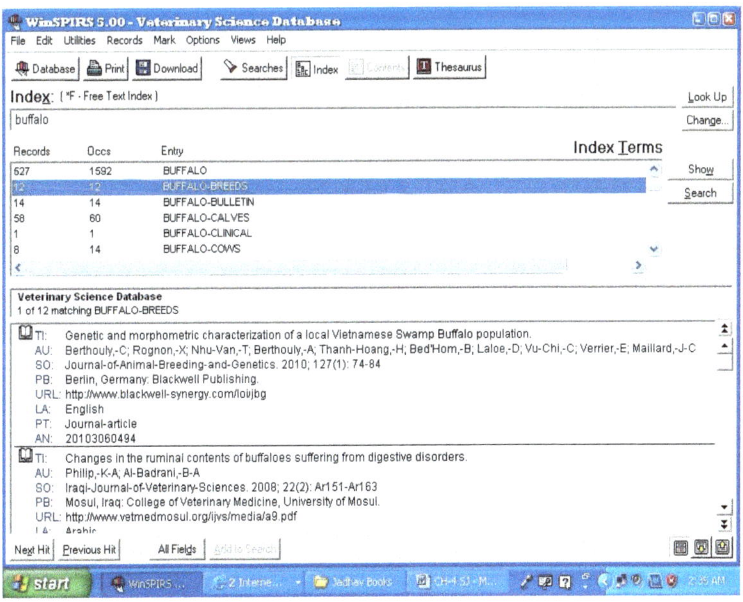

Handbooks

Handbooks are the compilations of miscellaneous information in a compact and handy manner. These are most frequently used by the scientists and technologists and form handy information in other fields as well. Handbooks may contain data, procedures, tables, graphs, diagrams and illustrations, etc. Handbooks and Manuals are another category of useful sources of ready reference type which are used by librarians in many libraries alive to user's queries. The word 'Hand book' is believed to have been derived from the German 'Handbook', and was first introduced in the 19th century. Handbook is said to be a small book or treatise, and as may conveniently be held in hand. Similarly, a Manual is also a book intended to b kept at hand for reference. In view of their features the two sources seem to be identical. They aim to bridge the gap between the normal textbook on theory and its practical application, thus facilitating economic and efficient practice.

- Bhatacharjee, S. K. (2000). Handbook of aromatic plants. Jaipur: Pointers Publications.
- Bhatacharjee, S. K.(2004). Handbook of medical plants (4th rev.ed.). Jaipur: Pointers Publications.
- Handbook on Minerals and mines in India. (2003). New Delhi: India Book Center.
- Bunch, B. (1996). Handbook of Current Science and Technology. Detroit: Gale Research.
- Sharma, R. P. (Ed.). (2001). Handbook of Agriculture. New Delhi: Indian Council of Agricultural Research.

Review of Progress

Reviews are critical in nature written by leading scientists in various focused disciplines providing clear picture about the current status and trends of development. Reviews of progress are prepared because the scanning of indexes and abstracts proves a cumbersome job for scientists and technologists. These provide an evaluative summary prepared by a specialist about the developments in a particular field over a given period. The reviews of progress are regarded as a pathway through the jungle of literature.

- Annual review of Astronomy and Astrophysics. (2000). Palo Alto, California: Annual Reviews.

- ☆ Annual review of Physiology. (2000). Palo Alto, California: Annual Reviews.
- ☆ Advances in Botanical research. (2000). New York: Academic Press.
- ☆ Annual review of Pathology. (2000). Palo Alto, California: Annual reviews.
- ☆ Progress in Neurobiology. (2000). Oxford: Elsevier Science.

2.2.3 Tertiary Sources

Primary sources have emerged as a medium to communicate original research. Due to increase in number primary sources resulted secondary sources and increase in number of secondary sources led to the tertiary sources. In other words, access to all the primary documents is impossible for a researcher. Therefore, to have the list of sources and location of information of these primary documents, a number of secondary documents are published and made available. Though secondary documents act as keys to primary documents, they themselves are also quite large in number, making it difficult to go through each and every one of them. Hence, the tertiary documents are used to locate secondary sources. Some of the tertiary sources are: directories, yearbooks, and bibliography of bibliographies.

Directories

Directories are the compilation of names and addresses arranged for reference purposes and are generally organized in alphabetical order. A directory may include indexes by subject field, geographical location, or some other desirable classification. These make up the largest single category of reference books. Some of the directories in the field of science and technology are:

- ☆ State-by-State Biotechnology directory. (1990). Rockville, Maryland: Biotechnology Information Institute.
- ☆ Biogeographical Society of Japan. Bulletin. (2000) Japan: Biogeographical Society of Japan.
- ☆ Federal Biotechnology transfer Directory. (2000). Rockville, Maryland: Biotechnology Information Institute.
- ☆ Information Industry Directory. (2000). Farmington Hills, Michigan: The Gale Group.
- ☆ Medical Company Guide to Japan. (2000). Japan: Chemical daily.

Yearbooks

Yearbooks are reference books which describe the events pertaining to a particular year. In various disciplines of science and technology, much of the task of digesting the developments of a year is performed by annual reviews of progress, and this function is performed by yearbooks as well. In this way they form an important source of information in the field. Some examples of yearbooks are:

- ☆ Butler, D. (Ed.). (2001). The Nature Yearbook of Science and Technology. U.K.: Nature publishing group.
- ☆ The World Competitiveness Yearbook. (1999). Switzerland: IMD.
- ☆ Yearbook of Clinical Microbiology. (2000). Boca Raton, FL: CRC Press.
- ☆ Yearbook of Physical Anthropology. (2000). Hoboken, NJ: John Wiley and Sons.
- ☆ Yearbook of Agricultural Statistics of Bangladesh. (2000). Bangladesh: Bureau of Statistics.

Bibliography of Bibliographies

The vast quantity of bibliographic information available makes it impossible for users to know the precise number and location of bibliographies available. Therefore it is necessary that there is some kind of control over bibliographies being published in different subjects. For almost every subject, a significantly large number of bibliographies have appeared. A bibliography of bibliographies serves this purpose to locate the bibliographies available in the subject. Some of the well-known bibliographies are:

- ☆ A Botanical Bibliography: A guide to bibliographic material applicable to Botany. (1970). Minneapolis, MN: Burgess.
- ☆ Basterman, T. (1971). Physical Sciences: A bibliography of bibliographies. Lanham, MD: Roman Littlefield.
- ☆ Ingles, E. (Ed.). (1994). Bibliography of Canadian bibliographies. Toronto: University of Toronto Press.
- ☆ Basterman, T. (1965-67). A World Bibliography of Bibliographies and of Bibliographical Catalogues, Calendars, Abstracts, Digests, Indexes and the like (4th ed.). Geneve: Societas Bibliographica.

☆ Tomey, A. F. (1977). A World Bibliography of Bibliographies, 1964-74. Lanham, MD: Roman and Littlefield.

References and Further Readings

Grogan, D. (1982). Science and Technology: An introduction to the literature (4th. ed.). London: Clive Bingley.

Saunderson, K. M. (1972). Patent as a source of technical information. *Aslib Proceedings,* 24, 244-254.

Singh, Sewa (2004). Manual of Reference and Information Source. Vols. 1 and 2. B R Publisher.

Chapter 3

Classification and Organization of Library Sources

3.1 Library Classification

Developments in our ability to store and retrieve large amounts of information have stimulated an interest in new ways to exploit this information for advancing human knowledge, which has resulted for classification. Systematic grouping of entities to meet one's requirement is known as classification. Classification lies at the root of all human activities. In fact, daily life is very much dependent on the process of classification, however, elementary this process may be. Classification is the process of organizing resources based on similar characteristics. The word classification was derived from the Latin word "classes" which meant order or rank of mobility in Roman society based upon birth and wealth. Classification is a mental process by which group or separate things are organised on the basis of common characteristics. In library science, classification refers to a systematic method of organizing library sources either books, serials, audiovisual materials, computer files etc., according to their subject by adopting some standard method of classification schemes like Colon Classification (CC), Dewey Decimal Classification (DDC), Universal Decimal Classification (UDC) and Library of Congress Classification (LCS), etc.

The complexity of thought content and the nature of relationships between various types of documents must be known and clearly established for their maximum use and is ensured by personal assistance to readers, systematic arrangement, and proper display of materials in the library. If the collection of a library is arranged in a systematic way, then the documents can be located and retrieved easily. The main purpose of library classification is to facilitate easy retrieval of documents in the library from the user perspectives and to facilitate pooling of collections on one subject at a central place.

According to Dr S.R. Ranganathan, Library classification aims to translate the subject into an ordinal number and individualization of a given document in the total order of documents in a library. The subject of the document is translated into a class number with the help of a notation. But, several documents are likely to bear the same class number and the problem of individualization arises. The class number is, therefore, not enough. It has to be supplemented by one or two, additional elements. These additional elements are book number and collection number. Class number, book number and collection number constitute the **call number** of a document.

Call Number = Class Number + Book Number + Collection Number

Ex: Applied Animals of Domestic Animals by R.L. Bharadwaj

According to Dewey Decimal Classification (DDC), Call Number is 636.0891 BHA (R)

636.0891 – **Class Number**

BHA – **Book Number** (Three letters of surname)

R – **Reference Book** (Type of Collections as reference and not for issue)

3.2 Major Schemes of Library Classification Schemes

3.2.1 Dewey Decimal Classification

Dewey Decimal Classification (**DDC**, also called the **Dewey Decimal System**) is a proprietary system of library classification developed by Melvil Dewey in 1876. It has been greatly modified and expanded through 22 major revisions, the most recent in 2003. This system organizes books on library shelves in a specific and repeatable order that makes it easy to find any book and return it to its proper place.

The Dewey Decimal Classification (DDC) system, devised by library pioneer Melvil Dewey in the 1870s provides a dynamic structure for the organization of library collections and is the world's most widely used library classification system. This is available in 22nd edition in print and online version. This scheme is organized into ten main classes and is very user friendly for both librarians and users of the library. Classification standards are available in print and Web formats, and full and abridged editions. The DDC provides meaningful notation in universally recognized Arabic numerals, well-defined categories and hierarchies, and a rich network of relationships among topics. This scheme of classification is updated at regular intervals to incorporate new subjects.

The DDC has a number for all books, including fiction: American fiction is classified in 813. Most libraries create a separate fiction section to allow shelving in a more generalized fashion than Dewey provides for, or to avoid the space that would be taken up in the 800s, or simply to allow readers to find preferred authors by alphabetical order of surname.

The system is made up of seven tables and ten main classes, each of which are divided into ten secondary classes or subcategories, each of which contain ten subdivisions.

The tables are:

- Standard subdivision
- Areas
- Subdivision of individual literatures
- Subdivisions of individual languages
- Racial, ethnic, national groups
- Languages
- Persons

The classes are:

- 000 – Computer science, information and general works
- 100 – Philosophy and psychology
- 200 – Religion
- 300 – Social sciences

- ☆ 400 – Language
- ☆ 500 – Science (including mathematics)
- ☆ 600 – Technology and applied Science
- ☆ 700 – Arts and recreation
- ☆ 800 – Literature
- ☆ 900 – History, geography, and biography

630 Agriculture and related technologies

631 Techniques, equipment and materials

632 Plant injuries, diseases and pests

633 Field and plantation crops

634 Orchards, fruits and forestry

635 Garden crops (Horticulture)

636 Animal husbandry

- 636.1 Equines and Horses
- 636.2 Ruminants and Camelidae Bovidae Cattle
- 636.3 Smaller Ruminants Sheep
- 636.4 Swine
- 636.5 Poultry Chickens
- 636.6 Birds other than poultry
- 636.7 Dogs
- 636.8 Cats
- 636.9 Other mammals

637 Processing dairy and related products

- 637.1 Milk Processing
- 637.2 Butter processing
- 637.3 Cheese processing
- 637.4 Manufacture of frozen desserts
- 637.5 Egg processing

638 Insect culture

639 Hunting, fishing and conservation

3.2.2 Colon Classification

Colon classification (CC) is a system of library classification developed by S. R. Ranganathan, which is based on the concept of facet analysis It was the first ever faceted or analytico-synthetic classification. The first edition was published in 1933. Since then six more editions have been published. It is especially used in libraries in India.

Its name "Colon classification" comes from the use of colons to separate facets in class numbers. However, many other classification schemes, some of which are completely unrelated, also use colons and other punctuation in various functions. They should not be confused with Colon classification. This included a major new development about the introduction of the PMEST (Personality, Matter, Energy, Space, Time) categories which help in organizing library collections. Each of the five types of facets is associated with different punctuations, *i.e.*,

- , (comma) = Personality
- ; (semi-colon) = Matter
- : (colon) = Energy
- . (Period) = Space
- '(apostrophe) = Time

***Example*: Transplanting Rice Seedlings in India in the Monsoon**

Agriculture - J(main class BS/BF)

Rice - Plant [1PI] - 381

Seedling - Organ [IP2] - 91

Transplanting - Action or energy [E] - D

India - S - pace [S] - 44

Monsoon - Time [T] - v

The class number is, J, 381, 91:D.44 'v

Treatment for Headaches

Medicine – L (BS/BF0

Head – Organ [1P1]

Disease – Property [MP]-4

Ache – Pain (part of the disease)-17

Treatment – Action [E]-6

Hence, the final class number is L, 18; 417:6

As an example, the subject "research in the cure of tuberculosis of lungs by x-ray conducted in India in 1950" results in a call number

L,45;421:6;253:f.44'N5

The components of this call number represent

Medicine, Lungs; Tuberculosis: Treatment; X-ray:Research.India'1950

Contents

Organization

The Colon Classification uses 42 main classes that are combined with other letters, numbers and marks in a manner resembling the Library of Congress Classification to sort a publication.

Facets

CC uses five primary categories, or facets, to further specify the sorting of a publication. Collectively, they are called *PMEST*:

, Personality

; Matter or property

: Energy

. Space

' Time

Classes

The following are the main classes of CC, with some subclasses, the main method used to sort the subclass using the PMEST scheme and examples showing application of PMEST.

z Generalia

1 Universe of Knowledge

2 Library Science

3 Book science

4 Journalism

B Mathematics

B1 Arithmetic

B13 Theory of numbers

B2 Algebra

B23 Algebraic equations

B25 Higher Algebra

B3 Analysis

B33 Differential Equations *[equation] , [degree] , [order] : [problem]*

B331,1,2:1 Numerical solutions (*:1*) of ordered (33*1*) linear (*,1*) second order (*,2*) differential equations

B37 Real Variables

B38 Complex Variables

B4 Other Methods

B6 Geometry

B7 Mechanics

B8 Physico-Mathematics

B9 Astronomical Mathematics

C Physics

C1 Fundamentals of Physics

C2 Properties of Matter

C3 Sound

C4 Heat

C5 Light and Radiation

C6 Electricity

C7 Magnetism

C8 Cosmic Hypothesis

D Engineering

E Chemistry

facets

:1 General Chemistry

:2 Physical Chemistry

:3 Analytical Chemistry

:33 Qualitative Chemistry

:34 Quantitative Chemistry

:35 Volumetric Chemistry

:4 Synthetic Chemistry

:5 Extraction Chemistry

E1 Inorganic Chemistry

E10 Group 0

E11 Group 1

E110 Hydrogen

E1109 Lithium

E111 Sodium

E2 Hydroxl (Base)

E3 Acid

E4 Salt

E5 Organic Substance

F Technology

G Biology

H Geology

H1 Mineralogy

H2 Petrology

H3 Structural Geology

H4 Dynamic Geology

H5 Stratigraphy

H6 Paleontology

H7 Economic Geology

H8 Cosmic Hypothesis

HX Mining

I Botany

J Agriculture

facets

:1 Soil

:3 Propagation

:4 Disease

:5 Development

:6 Breeding

:7 Harvest

:91 Nomenclature

:92 Morphology

:93 Physiology

:95 Ecology

material facets

,2 Bulb

,3 Root

,4 Stem

,5 Leaf

,6 Flower

,7 Fruit

,8 Seed

,97 Whole Plant

J1 Horticulture

J2 Feed

J3 Food

J4 Stimulant

J5 Oil

J6 Drug

J7 Fabric

J8 Dye

K Zoology *(same facet schedule as I Botany)*

KZ Animal Husbandry *(same facet schedule as I Botany)*

L Medicine *[organ]:[problem],[cause]:[handling]*

LZ3 Pharmacology *[substance].[action],[organ]*

LZ5 Pharmacopoeia

M Useful arts

M7 Textiles *[material]:[work]*

D Spiritual experience and mysticism *[religion],[entity]:[problem]*

N Fine arts

NA Architecture *[style] , [utility] , [part] : [technique]*

ND Sculpture *[style] , [figure] ; [material] : [technique]*

NN Engraving

NQ Painting *[style] , [figure] ; [material] : [technique]*

NR Music *[style] , [music] ; [instrument] : [technique]*

O Literature

P Linguistics

Q Religion

R Philosophy

S Psychology

T Education

U Geography

V History

W Political science

X Economics

Y Sociology

Z Law

Example

The most commonly cited example of the Colon Classification is the classification for:

- "Research in the cure of the tuberculosis of lungs by x-ray conducted in India in 1950s":
- Main classification is Medicine
  - (Medicine)
- Within Medicine, the Lungs are the main concern
  - (Medicine, Lungs)
- The property of the Lungs is that they are afflicted with Tuberculosis
  - (Medicine, Lungs; Tuberculosis)
- The Tuberculosis is being performed (:) on, that is the intent is to cure (Treatment)
  - (Medicine, Lungs; Tuberculosis: Treatment)
- The matter that we are treating the Tuberculosis with are X-Rays
  - (Medicine, Lungs; Tuberculosis: Treatment; X-ray)
- And this discussion of treatment is regarding the Research phase
  - (Medicine, Lungs; Tuberculosis: Treatment; X-ray: Research)
- This Research is performed within a geographical space (.) namely India
  - (Medicine, Lungs; Tuberculosis: Treatment; X-ray: Research.India)

- ☆ During the time (') of 1950
    - o (Medicine, Lungs; Tuberculosis: Treatment; X-ray: Research.India'1950)
- ☆ And translating into the codes listed for each subject and facet the classification becomes
    - o L,45;421:6;253:f.44'N5

3.2.3 Universal Decimal Classification

The **Universal Decimal Classification** is a system of library classification developed by the Belgian bibliographers Paul Otlet and Henri La Fontaine at the end of the 19th century. It is based on the Dewey Decimal Classification, but uses auxiliary signs to indicate various special aspects of a subject and relationships between subjects. It thus contains a significant faceted or analytico-synthetic element, and is used especially in specialist libraries. UDC has been modified and extended through the years to cope with the increasing output in all disciplines of human knowledge, and is still under continuous review to take account of new developments.

The documents classified by UDC may be in any form. They will often be literature, *i.e.* written documents, but may also be in other media such as films, video and sound recordings, illustrations, maps, and realia such as museum pieces.

UDC classifications use Arabic numerals and are based on the decimal system. Every number is thought of as a decimal fraction with the initial decimal point omitted, which determines filing order. For ease of reading, a UDC identifier is usually punctuated after every third digit. Thus, after 61 "Medical sciences" come the subdivisions 611 to 619; under 611 "Anatomy" come its subdivisions 611.1 to 611.9; under 611.1 come all of its subdivisions before 611.2 occurs, and so on; after 619 comes 620. An advantage of this system is that it is infinitely extensible, and when new subdivisions are introduced, they need not disturb the existing allocation of numbers.

The Main Categories

- ☆ 0 generalities
- ☆ 1 philosophy, psychology
- ☆ 2 religion, theology
- ☆ 3 social sciences

- 4
- 5 natural sciences
- 6 technology
- 7 the arts
- 8 language, linguistics, literature
- 9 geography, biography, history

A document may be classified under a combination of different categories through the use of additional symbols. For example:

Symbol	*Symbol Name*	*Meaning*	*Example*
+	plus	addition	*e.g.* 59+636 zoology and animal breeding
/	stroke	extension	*e.g.* 592/599 Systematic zoology (everything from 592 to 599 inclusive)
:	colon	relation	e.g. 17:7 Relation of ethics to art
[]	square brackets	algebraic subgrouping	*e.g.* 311:[622+669](485) statistics of mining and metallurgy in Sweden (the auxiliary qualifies 622+669 considered as a unit)
=	equals	language	*e.g.* =111 in English; 59=111 Zoology, in English

The Universal Decimal Classification (UDC) is a classification scheme for all fields of knowledge, a sophisticated indexing and retrieval tool. It was adapted by Paul Otlet and Nobel Prizewinner Henri La Fontaine from the Decimal Classification of Melvil Dewey, and first published (in French) between 1904 and 1907. It is well suited to indexing non-traditional media, multi-media collections, motion pictures, map collections, art collections and web-based directories of learning resources. UDC is a highly flexible and effective system for organizing bibliographic records for all kinds of information in any medium. UDC's most innovative and influential feature is its ability to express not just simple subjects but relations between subjects. This facility is added to a hierarchic structure, in which knowledge is divided into ten classes, then each class is subdivided into its logical parts, each subdivision is further subdivided, and so on. The two kinds of tables in UDC are main tables *i.e.* 'schedules' and auxiliary tables called 'common auxiliary tables'. The sample of UDC schedule for Agriculture and Animal Husbandry are:

Main Table

6 Applied sciences. Medicine. Technology

600 Technology

610 Medicine and health

611 Medicine

612 Pharmacy

613 Biomedical Sciences

614 Public Health

615 Kinesitherapy - Physical Training

620 Engineering. Technology in general

620 Materials testing. Commercial materials. Power stations. Economics of energy

621 Mechanical engineering in general. Nuclear technology. Electrical engineering. Machinery

621.3 Electrical engineering

622 Mining

623 Military engineering

624 Civil and structural engineering in general

625 Civil engineering and land transport. Railway engineering. Highway engineering

626 Hydraulic engineering in general

627 Natural waterway, port, harbour and shore engineering. Navigational, dredging, salvage and rescue facilities. Dams and hydraulic power plant

628 Public health engineering. Water. Sanitation. Illuminating engineering

629 Transport vehicle engineering

630 Agriculture

640 Home and family management

650 Management and public relations

660 Chemical engineering

670 Manufacturing

680 Manufacture for specific uses

690 Building and construction

6 APPLIED SCIENCES. MEDICINE, TECHNOLOGY

- **60** Biotechnology
- **61** Medical sciences
- **62** Engineering. Technology in general
- **63** Agriculture and related sciences and techniques. Forestry. Farming. Wildlife exploitation
  - **630** Forestry
    - **630*0** Forests, forestry and the utilization of forest products
    - **630*1** Factors of the environment. Forest biology
    - **630*2** Silviculture
    - **630*3** Work science (work studies) in forestry. Harvesting of wood: logging and transport. Forest engineering
    - **630*4** Forest injuries and protection
    - **630*5** Forest mensuration. Increment, development and structure of stands. surveying and mapping
    - **630*6** Forest management. Business economics of forestry.
    - Administration and organization of forest enterprises
    - **630*7** Marketing of forest products. Economics of forest transport and the wood industries
    - **630*8** Forest products and their utilization
    - **630*9** Forests and forestry from the national point of view. Social economics of forestry

- ⊞ **631/635** Farm management. Agronomy. Horticulture
- ⊟ **636** Animal husbandry and breeding in general. Livestock rearing. Breeding of domestic animals
  - ⊞ **636.01/.09** Special auxiliary numbers for animal husbandry
  - **636.1** Domestic equines. Horses
  - **636.2** Large ruminants. Cattle, oxen
  - **636.3** Small ruminants
  - **636.4** Pigs. Swine
  - **636.5** Poultry
  - **636.6** Birds (except poultry and game) bred or kept by humans
  - **636.7** Dogs
  - **636.8** Cats
  - **636.9** Other animals kept by humans
- **637** Produce of domestic (farmyard) animals and game
- **638** Keeping, breeding and management of insects and other arthropods
- ⊞ **639** Hunting, Fishing, Fish breeding

3.3 Role of Classification in the Internet Era

The Library is a storehouse of knowledge committed to serve the society at large, as temple of learning providing high quality information resources to support the academic and research endeavor. The success of any information system depends not merely on the quality of information resources but how well it is organized to provide access to the document collection. The techniques of traditional classification schemes play a significant role in the organization of information that aids retrieval in a network environment especially the Internet.

Emergence of Information and Communication technologies mainly the Internet and the World Wide Web (WWW) for the storage and retrieval of avalanche of information has changed the perception of classification. Due to the enormous growth of networked resources on the Internet, finding the relevant information has become a serious problem to the users. Thanks to the classification tools, may not be in toto, but the idea has been borrowed and implemented to bridge the gap. An approach developed for searching information on the Internet has been through search engines, which could be used for powerful keyword searches, although it has a tendency to come out with huge irrelevant information. While the other approach is producing 'Hot-lists' which would encourage users to browse the WWW. The techniques of library classification schemes has been employed in many of the search engines especially subject search engines to provide the subject hierarchy has encouraged the users to browse the Internet for information. A good example is **Yahoo** (http://www.yahoo.com) devised their own classification scheme providing structured hierarchical access to the resources.

The classification schemes provided a great boon offering solutions by providing improved access to World Wide Web resources. Web sites have been created to act as a hyper-guide to other web sites selected according to some pre-specified criteria and some of these sites typically consist of an alphabetical list of subjects, and selected Web resources.

3.3.1 Classifications and Internet

The potential of library classification techniques and tools have been realized to improve subject retrieval of pertinent information. However, it should be noted that much of the renewed interest in classification as an organizing and retrieval device for information resources has been sparked by the growth in usage of the Internet and World Wide Web (WWW). Koch, T (1998) stated that classification systems are used increasingly for organizing and retrieving information from the Internet as it gives advantages of well known, logical hierarchic structures as navigation support, but disadvantages, sometimes, of illogicality [1].

The uses of classification in online retrieval systems, includes to improve precision or recall; provide context for search terms, enable browsing, and to serve as a mechanism for switching between languages. The computerization of the DDC began with the production of DDC 19 (1979) from computer-based photocomposition

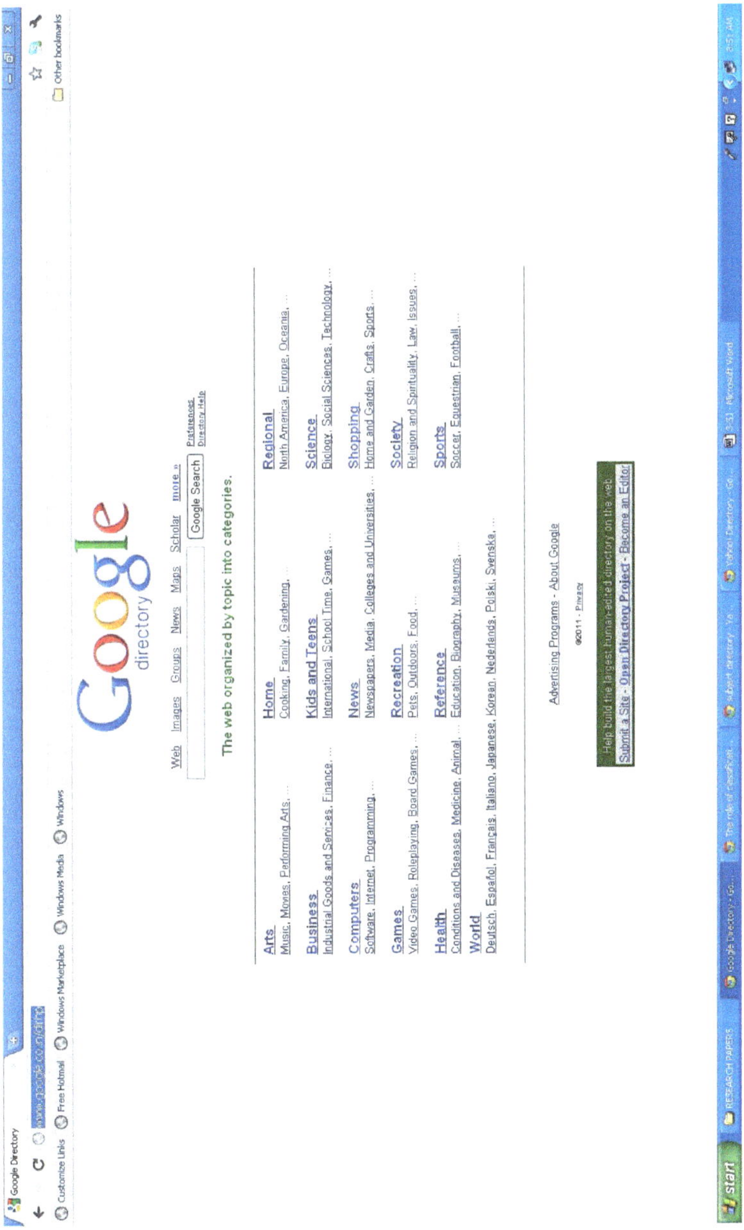
Google Directory
Google directory
Web Images Groups News Maps Scholar more »
Google Search
Preferences
Directory Help
The web organized by topic into categories.
Arts
Music, Movies, Performing Arts, ...
Home
Cooking, Family, Gardening, ...
Regional
North America, Europe, Oceania, ...
Business
Industrial Goods and Services, Finance, ...
Kids and Teens
International, School Time, Games, ...
Science
Biology, Social Sciences, Technology, ...
Computers
Software, Internet, Programming, ...
News
Newspapers, Media, Colleges and Universities, ...
Shopping
Home and Garden, Crafts, Sports, ...
Games
Video Games, Roleplaying, Board Games, ...
Recreation
Pets, Outdoors, Food, ...
Society
Religion and Spirituality, Law, Issues, ...
Health
Conditions and Diseases, Medicine, Animal, ...
Reference
Education, Biography, Museums, ...
Sports
Soccer, Equestrian, Football, ...
World
Deutsch, Español, Français, Italiano, Japanese, Korean, Nederlands, Polski, Svenska, ...
Advertising Programs - About Google
©2011 - Privacy
Help build the largest human-edited directory on the web
Submit a Site - Open Directory Project - Become an Editor
start

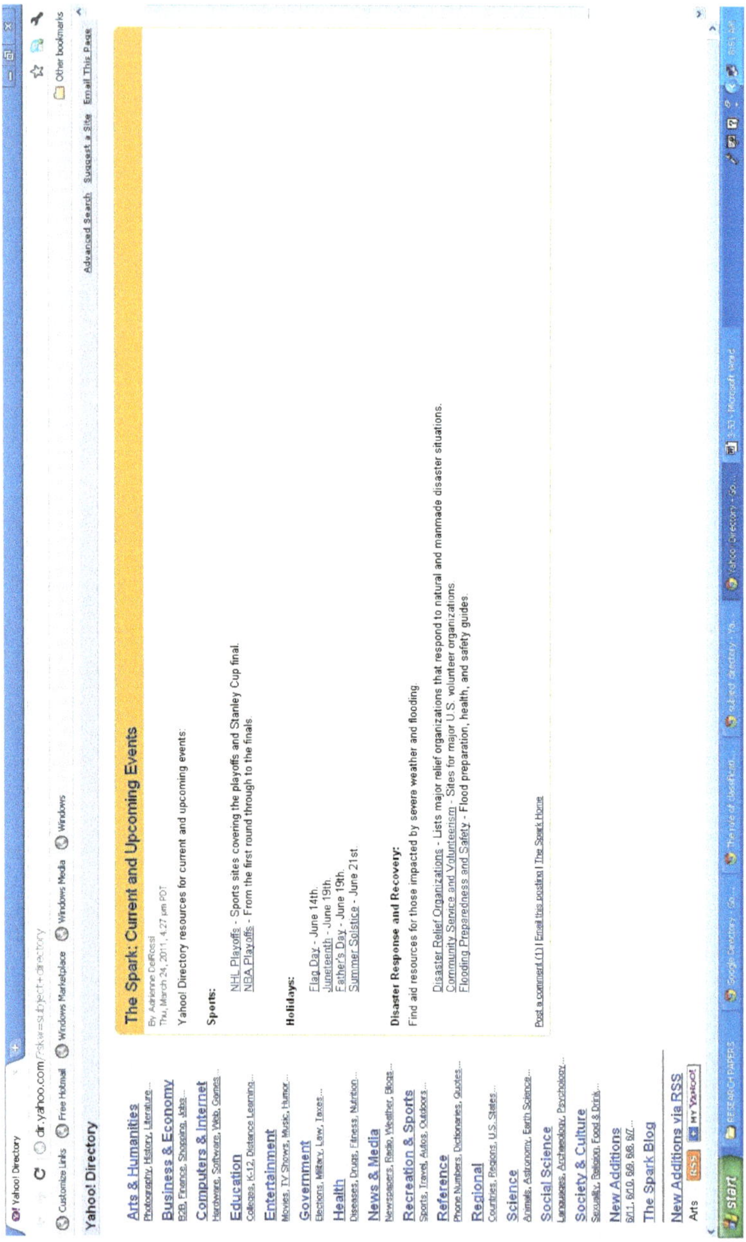
Yahoo! Directory
dir.yahoo.com/?skw=subject+directory
Customize Links
Free Hotmail
Windows Marketplace
Windows Media
Windows
Other bookmarks
Yahoo! Directory
Advanced Search
Suggest a Site
Email This Page
Arts & Humanities
Photography, History, Literature...
Business & Economy
B2B, Finance, Shopping, Jobs...
Computers & Internet
Hardware, Software, Web, Games...
Education
Colleges, K-12, Distance Learning...
Entertainment
Movies, TV Shows, Music, Humor...
Government
Elections, Military, Law, Taxes...
Health
Diseases, Drugs, Fitness, Nutrition...
News & Media
Newspapers, Radio, Weather, Blogs...
Recreation & Sports
Sports, Travel, Autos, Outdoors...
Reference
Phone Numbers, Dictionaries, Quotes...
Regional
Countries, Regions, U.S. States...
Science
Animals, Astronomy, Earth Science...
Social Science
Languages, Archaeology, Psychology...
Society & Culture
Sexuality, Religion, Food & Drink...
New Additions
6/11, 6/10, 6/9, 6/8, 6/7...
The Spark Blog
New Additions via RSS
Arts
RSS
MY YAHOO!
The Spark: Current and Upcoming Events
By Adrienne DelRossi
Thu, March 24, 2011, 4:27 pm PDT
Yahoo! Directory resources for current and upcoming events:
Sports:
NHL Playoffs - Sports sites covering the playoffs and Stanley Cup final.
NBA Playoffs - From the first round through to the finals.
Holidays:
Flag Day - June 14th.
Juneteenth - June 19th.
Father's Day - June 19th.
Summer Solstice - June 21st.
Disaster Response and Recovery:
Find aid resources for those impacted by severe weather and flooding.
Disaster Relief Organizations - Lists major relief organizations that respond to natural and manmade disaster situations.
Community Service and Volunteerism - Sites for major U.S. volunteer organizations.
Flooding Preparedness and Safety - Flood preparation, health, and safety guides.
Post a comment (1) | Email this posting | The Spark Home
start
RESEARCH PAPERS
Google Directory - Go...
The role of classificati...
subject directory - Ya...
Yahoo! Directory - Go...
Microsoft Word

tapes and in 1984 developed an online editorial support system (ESS) for the Dewey Classification resulting to produce DDC 20 (1989), the first classification to be produced using an online editorial support system.

A different path is being taken in the conversion of the LCC to machine-readable form. Recognizing the benefits of online classification data for maintenance and distribution of LCC, the Library of Congress began developing the USMARC Format for Classification Data in 1987. The format was given provisional approval in 1990 and shortly afterward the Library of Congress began converting the forty-six LCC schedules. Some of the websites provide users the ability to perform word or phrase searches to retrieve items of interest viz., Yahoo, Google and Infoseek, providing the additional capability of allowing users to navigate through a series of subject categories to discover potentially relevant documents. Although, these search engines use essentially the same input as the basis for their subject structures, the resulting categories displayed to users are quite different. The broad subject "Education" is found at the top level of both Yahoo and Infoseek, however, the next level under area "Education" reveals a very different organization of the topic in each system. In Yahoo (http:// dir.yahoo.com/) over 30 sub-categories are available for browsing education-related topics while Google presents a leaner outline (http://www.google.co.in/dirhp).

Library classification schemes have long provided a similar organizing tool for library materials. The subject categories found in the DDC and LCC are based largely on the topics expressed in monographic material in traditional book format. For printed books, the Dewey Summaries (http://www.oclc.org/fp/) and LC Classification Outline are the library community's functional equivalent to the subject categories of Yahoo and Infoseek. In fact, several noncommercial WWW sites are using DDC and LCC to provide subject access to Web-accessible documents. The first practical universal classification schemes were developed in the late-nineteenth-century for organising libraries in the context of rapidly growing knowledge and an increase in the numbers of printed books. The most widely-used universal classification schemes are Dewey Decimal Classification (DDC), the Universal Decimal Classification (UDC) and Library of Congress classification scheme (LCC). Use of a universal, multidisciplinary classification scheme in an Internet context results in retrieval of information and enables improved browsing and subject searching across services and collections from different subject areas. It is therefore subject specific classification schemes should be used to describe Internet resources for accessibility.

Use of Classification Schemes in Internet Search Resources

Dewey Decimal System (DDC)

The Dewey Decimal Classification System (DCC) was first produced by Melvil Dewey in 1876 originally produced for small American college library and currently in its 21st edition is used in the national bibliographies of the UK, Canada, Australia, Italy and other countries. Research carried out by OCLC in the 1980s established that DDC was a suitable tool for browsing, first for library catalogues and then for the Internet. The DDC has been widely used for organizing information on the Internet may not be in complete aspect but at least they have borrowed the techniques and tools for organization to provide information access.

More libraries than any other classification scheme available in the world have used DDC scheme of classification widely. It is currently used in 135 different countries and has been translated into 30 languages[2]. The Library of Congress Cataloguing Service in the bibliographic records it creates, along with the Library of Congress Classification Scheme (LCC) uses it. It appears in the Cataloguing in Publication data produced by the Library of Congress, the British Library and some other national libraries. OCLC has now taken over DDC and available at: URL:http://www.oclc.org/oclc/fp/fptxthm.htm

DDC 21st edition saw a major revision of the life sciences in 560-590 which saw a move away from the organism centred approach in earlier versions of DDC towards an orientation concentrating more upon processes and this scheme is updated more frequently than other classification schemes in the globe.

DDC 21st edition numbers of the first 3 digits are made is available on the Internet at: [http://www.oclc.org/oclc/fp/ddc/ddcsum21/ddc21sm1.htm] with the intention of supporting and encouraging library professionals, classifiers and other relevant personnel to use DDC to classify materials on the Internet. The software system Dewey for Windows is available on CD-ROM and however tools like this and the *Classification Plus* component of *Cataloger's Desktop* are only designed to give cataloguer's access to DDC and are not suitable for the application of DDC in an Internet environment.

OCLC's Net First Internet database includes Dewey Decimal Classification (DDC) numbers and Library of Congress subject headings to facilitate access to resources. Three OCLC research projects are helping explore the potential of DDC as a knowledge-structuring tool for large collections of electronic documents.

McKiernan (1996) lists 14 sites that use, or claim to use, Dewey Decimal Classification System (DDC) for the organization of resources [5]

Basalt Regional Library Homepage. Basalt, Colo.: Basalt Regional Library. <URL:http://www.colosys.net/basaltlib/>

Blue Web'n Content Categories. San Diego, Calif.: Pacific Bell. <URL:http://www.kn.pacbell.com/wired/bluewebn/categories.html>

Canadian Information by Subject. Ottawa: National Library of Canada.<URL:http://www.nlc-bnc.ca/caninfo/esub.htm>

CyberDewey: a Catalogue for the World Wide Web. David A Mundie (Pittsburgh, Penn.). <URL:http://ivory.lm.com/~mundie/DDHC/CyberDewey.html>

GNOSIS (Global Network Of Silicon Information Services). Patrick W. Clancey (Sun Microsystems). <URL:http://www.aimnet.com/~clancey/gnosis/>

The Internet Resource. Edinburgh: Napier University Library. <URL:http://www.napier.ac.uk/depts/library/intres/ir000999.html>

Internet Resources in Dewey Decimal Order with DDC Subjects. Independence, Mo.: Mid-Continent Public Library <URL:http://www.mcpl.lib.mo.us/dewey.htm>

Mr. Dui's Topic Finder. Dublin, Ohio: OCLC Office of Research. <URL:http://www.oclc.org/oclc/fp/mrdui/mrdui.htm>

Net Sites by the Numbers Tempe, Ariz.:Tempe Public Library. <URL:http://www.tempe.gov/library/bnindex.htm>

Sites by DDC. Alastair G. Smith (Victoria University of Wellington, New Zealand). <URL:http://www.vuw.ac.nz/~agsmith/bkmark.htm#ddc>

WEBrary(tm) (Online Ready Reference System). Morton Grove, Ill.: Morton Grove Public Library. <URL:http://www.nslsilus.org/mgkhome/orrs/webrary.html>

World Wide Web Reference Collection. Denton, Tex.: University of North Texas, School of Library and Information Sciences <URL:http://www-lan.unt.edu/slis/student/projects/wwwrc/Index.htm>

WWLib Browse Interface (Wolverhampton Web Library). Peter Burden (University of Wolverhampton, UK) <URL:http://www.scit.wlv.ac.uk/wwlib/browse.html>

Expanding Universe. Toronto, Ontario: Metropolitan Toronto Reference Library. <URL:http://www.mtrl.toronto.on.ca/centres/bsd/astronomy/index.html>

PICK: Quality Internet Resources in Library and Information Science Aberystwyth: University of Wales Aberystwyth, Thomas Parry Library. URL:http://www.aber.ac.uk/~tplwww/e/pick.html

Two further Internet sites that use DDC are *NetFirst* and *Biz/ed*:

NetFirst. Dublin, Ohio: OCLC. URL:http://www.oclc.org/oclc/netfirst/

NetFirst has used DDC to organise a browsing structure since October 1996. DDC notations had been present in their links from the start of the service, but have only recently been made available for browsing (Oehler 1996).

Biz/ed. Bristol: University of Bristol, Institute for Learning and Research Technology URL:http://www.bized.ac.uk/

Biz/ed is a subject service for business education, based at the University of Bristol and funded by a consortium of commercial and educational organizations, including Elib. *Biz/ed* offers an online catalogue of good quality Internet resources (using the ROADS software, and based on the *SOSIG* model - in fact, *SOSIG* and *Biz/ed* share the same offices). Since its inception in 1996, this catalogue has used an abridged version of DDC to classify resources, and to create browsable subject sections.

Universal Decimal Classification (UDC)

The Universal Decimal Classification (UDC) is an international scheme attempts to cover all areas of knowledge and its origins lie in the Dewey Decimal Classification adapted in end of the Nineteenth century by Paul Otlet and Henri LaFontaine in order to create a universal bibliography. UDC is an international standard, a widely recognized and used classification scheme and its structure allows composite codes to be assigned to provide complex and detailed description of the subject content of a document. The scheme consists of 60,000 classes (divisions and sub-divisions) as well as a number of auxiliary tables.

The abridged versions of UDC with a list of Classification numbers are available on the Internet to assist the library professionals and other persons to encourage and support organization of information on the net. The Intute has a selected classification numbers of UDC is available at [URL: http://www.intute.ac.uk/].

The Universal Decimal Classification (UDC) has been used in Internet Services. Some of the Internet services currently using UDC are:

BUBL

The BUBL Subject Tree aims to provide comprehensive UK Internet resources in all subject areas. The original Subject Tree of BUBL uses UDC, but it should be noted that *BUBL* is in the process of transforming into a new service called LINK that will be using the Dewey Decimal Classification Scheme. BUBL do not classify individual items, but do use the UDC to provide browsable sections for each subject area.

GERHARD

GERHARD (German Harvest Automated Retrieval and Directory), a funded project in the Deutsche Forchungsgemeinschaft The UDC is used in the enlarged and multilingual version of the ETH library Zürich aims to establish a service for searching and browsing German Internet resources by matching UDC entries by computer linguistic algorithms to create an searchable index and an automatically generated subject tree.

NISS

The NISS Directory of Networked Resources uses UDC and its hierarchies, with the numbers displayed on the screen, above each section. The Directory may be browsed in UDC number "inverted tree structure", UDC number linear structure (shelf order) or alphabetical subject heading order. NISS do not normally classify beyond the decimal point, although there are exceptions in the 'computing' and 'geography' sections.

OMNI

OMNI (Organizing Medical Networked Information) is a selective subject service that catalogues resources relating to medicine and uses UDC to create browsable sections. However, they also use a subject-based classification scheme, the NLM, which is used to create separate browsing sections. OMNI currently classify in as much detail as possible with the NLM scheme, but find this more difficult with the UDC scheme.

Intute (earlier SOSIG)

Intute remains a free online service, providing users with access to the very best Web resources for education and research, evaluated and selected by a network of subject specialists (http:// www.intute.ac.uk/). Intute is a free online service that helps you to find web resources for studies and research covers four new subject groups *i.e.* Science, Engineering and Technology (including geography), Arts and Humanities, Social Sciences and Health and Life Sciences. A selection of 26 UDC numbers is currently used for the browsing sections and in cataloguing however, a larger list is used.

Library of Congress Classification System (LCC)

One of the world's most widely spread classification schemes is the Library of Congress Classification System (LCC).LCC is used extensively in the United States, Canada and Australia, especially in academic and research and LCC notations are present in many records in OCLC (Online Computer Library Centre) and RLIN (Research Libraries Information Network). Since LCC is a general classification scheme it is likely to be less detailed in specific subjects than subject specific schemes. There are no examples of services using LCC for the classification of resources within a single subject area, like subject based information gateways.

The Library of Congress has developed a USMARC Format for Classification Data which allows classification data to interact with other USMARC bibliographic data and authority files. The format has been designed for use with DDC and LCC, (the two major classification systems used in the US), but permits communication with other classification schemes, especially UDC and NLM.

Some of the important Internet services, which make use of Library of Congress Classification system for classification of resources available on the Internet, are briefed below.

Cyberstacks

CyberStacks available at [URL:http://www.public.iastate.edu/~CYBERSTACKS] is a centralized, integrated, and unified collection of Internet resources categorized using the Library of Congress classification scheme.

The WWW Virtual Library

The WWW Virtual Library is a quite comprehensive subject catalogue making use of LCC system. All the main classes in the LCC system are represented and this WWW Virtual Library does not use the classification notations themselves at all in their LCC structure but uses only their corresponding headings. It is accessed at http://www.w3.org/pub/DataSources/bySubject/LibraryOf Congress.html. The two libraries trying to organize Internet resources in accordance with LCC are Cardinal Stritch College Library and Seattle Pacific University Library- Subject Oriented Resources.

References and Further Readings

Ardo, A., Falcoz, F., Koch, T., Nielsen, M., Sandfaer, M., (1994). Improving resource discovery and retrieval on the Internet. The Nordic WAIS/World Wide Web Project - Summary report. *NORDINFO Nytt*, 4, 13-28. URL:http://www.ub2.lu.se/W4/ summary.html

Khanna, J.K. (1986). *Colon Classification.* New Delhi, India: Ess Ess Publications.

Koch,T. (1998).The use of classification systems for improved description, organisation and search of Internet resources. *Buch-und-Bibliothek,* 50 (5) May, p. 326-32, 35.

Koch, T. and Day, M. (1997). The role of classification schemes in Internet resource description and discovery, *DESIRE* D3.2 (3), February. http://www.ukoln.ac.uk/metadata/desire/classification/

Krishan Kumar (1988). Theory of Classification, 4th ed. New Delhi: Vikas Publishing.

Kumar, P.S.G. (1987). *Introduction to Colon Classification, Edition 7.* Nagpur, India: Dattsons,

Marcella, Rita and Newton, Robert (1996). A New Manual of Classification. New Delhi: Jaico Publishing.

Mills, J. (1996). A Modern Outline of Library Classification. Bombay: Asia Publishing.

McKiernan, G., (1996). *Beyond bookmarks: schemes for organizing the Web.* URL:http://www.iastate.edu/~CYBERSTACKS/CTW.htm

Ohedar, A.K. and B. Sengupta (1977). Library Classification, 2nd rev. ed. Calcutta: World Press.

Parkhi, R.S.(1964). *Decimal Classification and Colon Classification in Perspective.* New York: Asia Publishing House.

Raju, A.A.N. (1984). *Decimal Universal Decimal and Colon Classification.* Delhi, India: Ajanta Publications.

Ranganathan, S. R. (1987). Colon Classification, 7th ed. Edited by M.A. Gopinath. Bangalore: Sarada Ranganathan Endowment for Library Science. 34 Elements of Library Classification.

Ranganathan, S.R. (1962). Elements of Library Classification, 3rd ed. Bombay: Asia Publishing.

Ranganathan, S.R. (1967). Prolegomena to Library Classification, 3rd ed. Bangalore: Sarada Ranganathan Endowment for Library Science.

Ranganathan, S.R.(1933). *Colon Classification.* Madras, India: Madras Library Association.

Satija, M.P. and Agrawal, S.P. (1996). Book Number- Some Indian Methods. 2nd edn. New Delhi: Reliance Publishing.

Shafer, K. (1996). *A brief introduction to Scorpion.* Dublin, Ohio: OCLC. URL:http://orc.rsch.oclc.org:6109/bintro.html

Thompson, R., Shafer, K. and Vizine-Goetz, D. (1997). *Evaluating Dewey concepts as a knowledge base for automatic subject assignment*. Dublin, Ohio: OCLC. URL:http://orc.rsch.oclc.org:6109/eval_dc.html

URL:http:// URL:http://www.niss.ac.uk/resource-description/udcbrief.html (Accessed on 02nd June, 2011).

www.oclc.org/oclc/fp/deweywin/dwytoc-t.htm (Accessed on 02nd June, 2011).

Vizine, Goetz.D. (1997). From book classification to knowledge organization: improving Internet resource description and discovery. Bulletin-of-the-American-Society-for-Information-Science. 24 (1) Oct/Nov. p.24-7.

Chapter 4

Veterinary Information Systems

4.1 Introduction

In the developing country like India animal husbandry plays a vital role in rural economy. It supplements household income especially for the landless, small and marginal farmers. It also provides subsidiary occupation in semi urban areas and for people living in hilly, tribal and draught-prone areas where crop output may not sustain the family. India is endowed with the largest livestock population in the world. As per livestock Census (2003), the country has about 18.5 crore cattle and 9.8 crore buffaloes which accounts for 14 percent of the cattle population and 57 percent of the worlds buffalo population. The contribution of livestock to total GDP has remained steady between 4.8 and 6.2 percent during the last two decades; and its contribution to agriculture GDP has gone up from 13.8 percent in 1981 to 23.8 percent in 2002-2003 (www. livestock census, 2003).

Veterinary education is the most potential instrument for the social change and development. India stands number one in milk production and fourth in poultry production in the global market. Animal husbandry as compared other agricultural products has several advantages, such as relative stability in yield and price, regular cash flow throughout the year, utilization of family labour, use of crop residues as cattle feed has helped in laying a stable foundation for rural development. The Indian animal husbandry industry has acquired substantial growth from the Eighth Plan onwards. Country ranks first in the world in milk production which accounts for 15 percent of the world's total milk production. Country's milk output has not only placed the dairy industry first in the world, but also represents sustained growth in the availability of milk and milk products. Milk is now the largest contributor to the National GDP contributing about 5.3% to India's agricultural GDP even larger than rice and wheat combined. The value of output from milk at current prices during 2006-07 has been over Rs. 144386 crore and contributes to nearly 70 percent of total livestock sector output. As many as 120 million rural families are engaged in animal husbandry (Pawar and Amrutkar, 2009).

A veterinarian (North America English) or a veterinary surgeon (British English) often shortened to "Vet" is an animal physician and practitioner of veterinary medicine. Veterinary Education is the study of veterinary science and its application in professional practice. The word veterinarian comes from the word "Veterinae" meaning "Draught animals". The word veterinarian was first used in English by Thomas Browne (1605-1692). Veterinary as an adjective is used for the one who have expertise in disease of domestic animals. (Singh, 2007).

4.2 Veterinary Education: Historical Perspective

Formal veterinary education began in the western world in the 1760s in Lyon and Alfort in France with the establishment of first western veterinary colleges. The French colleges had high standards for producing well educated veterinarians who quickly addressed important animal health problems of the day and the new profession flourished. The first Anglophone College was established in London in 1791. The first successful colleges in North America were private institutions modeled after British Veterinary colleges. The New York Veterinary College established in 1857 and the Ontario Veterinary College in 1862.

Between the World Wars, veterinary education in the United States was consolidated in the land-grant colleges. The land-grant tradition of teaching, research, and public service was adopted by veterinary colleges. Veterinary education, however, was poorly supported during this period, which reflected the lack of public concern for the profession.

Veterinary education in India can be traced between pre-independence and post independence period.

Pre-Independence Period

History of animal science education in India begins with the domestication of animals. Though animal science education in the broad sense includes education in Veterinary science, Animal husbandry, Dairying and Fisheries, very little information is available on the ancient history of education in dairy and fisheries science. Domestication of animals is said to have been started in India during the neolithic age evidenced from the paintings in the potteries and the bones of the animals discovered during excavations in the sites of early civilization. The goat was the first ruminant to be domesticated and the horse the last, as late in 2000 BC in countries near middle- east.

In Indian subcontinent, Veterinary education is as old as human civilization. *Salhotra* from the vedic period was considered as the *"Father of Veterinary Science"*, an expertise in treating diseases of horse, elephant and cow. He wrote "Asvayueveda Sidhayoga Samgraha (Haya Ayurveda)" which was considered a standard equine therapy book. This is the reason, in earlier times the veterinarian was called as *Salutri*. *Sushrut* son of *Salihotra* was also a renound surgeon and hundreds of surgical instrument suggested by him are still used in modern surgery. "Palakapya" a contemporary of Salhotra wrote "Hasthy ayurveda" a book on elephant treatment. Among pandavas, Nakula wrote "Asva Chikitsa" (Horse treatment) and "Vaidyaka Sarvasva" (Medicine) and Sahadeva wrote "Gosastra" on cattle.

During the Mauryan age (322 to 232 BC), there were superintendents of cows responsible to supervise herds of milch cows, calves, work of herdsmen, milkers, churners, hunters and also to look after stored milk and ghee (Arvindan, 2002). During the reign of king Ashoka, veterinary hospitals were established in the state institutions. In this period, though there is evidence of state-run veterinary hospitals, there is no mention on the mode of training of the Veterinarians. However, it can be presumed that earlier veterinary education was imparted by the states to their disciples. Further information on veterinary science is available from the early period of British rule in India.

During pre-independence period, veterinary science does not seem to have received much attention till the end of 18th century, when the East India Company recognized the need to improve the quality of horses and bullocks for its military power.

To meet their military needs, some horse-breeding farms were started in 1774 in the army establishments. These stud farms were looked after by men from England. No Indian Veterinarian was available till 1783 when the army authorities became extremely worried about the rapid prevalence of equine diseases. Though the services of a few specialists were made available to the army by 1799, no information is available about their professional background. Willium Moorcraft, however, has been a distinguished figure in this regard who after his medical career had received training at the Veterinary School at Lyons, France. The first training course in veterinary science was organized in 1821 by Dr. J. T. Hodgson, who was the veterinary surgeon to the Governor-General's Bodyguard in Calcutta, to train persons to be employed as sub-assistant veterinary surgeons with corps of Indian cavalry (Arvindan, 2002).

These activities lead to the establishment of an army veterinary department in India in 1827. A beginning in the formal education in veterinary science was made in the country in 1862, when a veterinary school was opened in Poona (Pune) mainly to train persons for the army veterinary department. Soon it was realized that attention should be paid to cattle population also since the diseases of cattle were spreading fast. This resulted in the appointment of Cattle Plague Commission in 1869. Some more veterinary schools came up subsequently, *viz.*, at Hapur in 1879, Ajmer in 1881 and Simla in 1888. Another veterinary school was set up in Bombay in 1886. Following frequent recurrence of famine and outbreaks of diseases, several commissions were set up towards the end of the 19th century to go in to the question of cattle plague, and preservation and maintenance of health of bullocks. With the expansion of the civil veterinary departments, necessity for more veterinary colleges arose. The Bengal veterinary college was opened in 1892 and the Madras veterinary college in 1902. A fourth institution was opened in Patna in 1930. Primary objective of the education programme was to create a cadre of veterinarians to look after the health problems of domestic animals, and to manage the dairy herds maintained by the military and Government farms.

Post-Independence Period

When the country attained independence in 1947, there were 6 colleges with an intake capacity of about 300 students. As a result of partition of the country, Lahore Veterinary College was transferred to Pakistan and in order to accommodate the displaced students, the Punjab Government started the Hisar Veterinary College in 1948. Accordingly emergency steps were taken for increasing the output of graduates by increasing the admission capacity through establishing new colleges, introducing double shift and also by instituting an emergency diploma programme of two year duration. More colleges were established at Assam and Jabalpur (1948), Bikaner (1954) Trichur, Tirupathi, Mhow and Bhubneshwar (1955). With these efforts admission capacity increased. In addition, an emergency diploma programme was started at Hisar, Uttar Pradesh, Bihar, West Bengal, Rajasthan, Madhya Pradesh, and Andhra Pradesh. The training programme was based on a model Syllabus developed by the Indian Council of Agricultural Education (ICAE) under the ICAR which was somewhere between those of stockman training course and regular degree programme giving emphasis to the practical training rather than theory. It was expected that those trained personnel's will be able to serve in the newly formed NES blocks as middle-level workers of animal husbandry, to undertake first-aid treatment of sick animals, undertake artificial insemination works related to animal husbandry. This move was also faced with some problems due to lack of minimum required qualification for admission to degree programme for some of the candidates. Finally through the intervention of the ICAR most of these candidates were re-admitted to colleges and condensed courses were conducted for completing their degree requirements.

During 1955-56, there were 14 colleges with an intake capacity of about 1,300 students. By 1960, number of colleges increased to 17, including the newly established Veterinary College at Pantnagar, under the UP Agricultural University, the first of its kind in the country. These are now 43 veterinary colleges in India offering composite programs in veterinary science and animal husbandry. The total intake of students in each college is around 60-70. Of the 42 colleges and one deemed university, 24 functions under Agricultural Universities; and 18 veterinary colleges functioning under the Universities of Veterinary Sciences in different parts of the states in India. It is imperative that, in a degree program in veterinary science, sufficient courses be offered to make the graduates competent for adequate animal health coverage but that, at the same time, sufficient courses in animal science be taught to make them competent to meet the challenges of rural- based livestock problems. After completing the courses in veterinary and animal husbandry, students are usually given internship training for a period of six months in both veterinary science and animal husbandry. This on site training gives them the confidence to face the problems of rural areas.

Post graduate training has been imparted to the veterinarians since 1900 at the Imperial Institute of Veterinary Research (IVRI). These training programmes were replaced by refresher courses in 1922. With the addition of newer departments of Animal Nutrition, Poultry Research, Animal Genetics etc. comprehensive training programmes were initiated in the following fields:

- ☆ Post-graduate refresher course in veterinary science (6 months duration)
- ☆ Advanced course in Poultry Husbandry (6 months duration)
- ☆ Advanced course in Animal Husbandry (8 months duration)
- ☆ A course on Manufacture of Sera and vaccines (9 months duration)
- ☆ Advanced course on Artificial Insemination and Physio-pathology of Reproduction (9 months duration)

Since 1942, in addition to these regular courses students have been admitted to associateship of IVRI (Indian Veterinary Research Institute, Barrielly), a diploma course of 2- year's duration. It consisted of research and training which was recognized as equivalent to post-graduate qualification for various jobs under central and state governments. Facilities for research and training at this institute were so immense that it has been recognized as a centre for post-graduate research and study leading to M.V.Sc and Ph.D. in as an institution for postgraduate studies leading to M.V.Sc and Ph.D. by the Madras University in 1936.

After independence of India, just very recently in 2000 "Post-graduate Institute of Veterinary and Animal Sciences", was established at Akola in Maharashtra state, which was recognized as post-graduate research institute leading only M.V. Sc. Degree programmes. Further, more veterinary colleges are in the offering the Post-graduation and research courses in different discipline of veterinary and animal sciences in many other states.

The objectives of a veterinarian in Indian context are:

- Animal health promotion.
- Primary veterinary science including animal husbandry *i.e.* promotion, prevention, rehabilitative and development services.
- Service rendered is effective – efficient affordable and acceptable to community.
- Involve in developing self-reliant-primitive system for good nutrition, good housing and health care through individuals or community involvement.
- Seek to promote development of animals through community so that animal and society are beneficial in complementary manner.

The Veterinary Council of India is a statutory body of the Government of India framed under an Act of Parliament *i.e.* Indian Veterinary Council Act, 1984 established with an objective

- To prepare and maintain the Indian Veterinary Practitioners' Register containing the names of all persons who possess the recognized veterinary qualifications and who are for the time being enrolled on a State Veterinary Register of the State to which Indian Veterinary Council Act extends.
- To lay down minimum standards of veterinary education required for granting recognized veterinary qualifications by veterinary institutions.
- To recommend recognition or withdrawal of recognition of veterinary qualifications granted by veterinary institutions in India.
- To lay down the standards of professional conduct, etiquette and code of ethics to be observed by veterinary practitioners.

- ☆ To negotiate with institutions located in other countries imparting training in veterinary education for recognition of their qualifications on reciprocal basis.
- ☆ To regulate veterinary practice in the country.
- ☆ To advise the Central and the State Governments on all regulatory matters concerning veterinary practice and education.
- ☆ To frame regulations and implement the provisions of the Act, and Rules and Regulations framed there under.

The Veterinary Colleges in India are established to enhance the livestock production, health improvements, milk production and strengthening the nation's wealth. Accordingly, Veterinary colleges have been contributing their share in upgrading the quality of veterinary education in the country through quality improvement of academic studies, and faculty improvement programmes. Presently there are 7 veterinary universities and 43 veterinary colleges. Out of 43 colleges, 18 are constituents of 7 state veterinary Universities and others are part of State Agricultural Universities (SAU's) and one is affiliated to general university (Pondicherry). The list of Veterinary Colleges in India is as under

List of Veterinary Colleges in India

Sl.No.	*Name of the Colleges*		*State*
1.	College of Veterinary Science	**Hyderabad**	Andhra Pradesh
2.	College of Veterinary Science	**Tirupati**	Andhra Pradesh
3.	N.T. Ramarao College of Veterinary Science	**Gannavram**	Andhra Pradesh
4.	College of Veterinary Science	**Guwahati**	Assam
5.	Lakhimpur College of Veterinary Science	**Lakhimpur**	Assam
6.	Bihar Veterinary College	**PATNA**	Bihar
7.	College of Veterinary Science and Animal Husbandry	**Durg**	Chattisgarh
8.	College of Veterinary Science and Animal Husbandry	**Anand**	Gujarat
9.	College of Veterinary Science and Animal Husbandry	**Sardar Krushinagar**	Gujarat

Contd...

Table–*Contd...*

Sl.No.	*Name of the Colleges*		*State*
10.	College of Veterinary Science	**Hissar**	Haryana
11.	College of Veterinary and Animal Sciences	**Palampur**	Himachal Pradesh
12.	College of Veterinary Sciences and Animal Husbandry	**Jammu**	Jammu and Kashmir
13.	College of Veterinary Sciences and Animal Husbandry	**Srinagar**	Jammu and Kashmir
14.	Ranchi College of Veterinary Science and Animal Husbandry	**Ranchi**	Jharkhand
15.	Veterinary College	**Bidar**	Karnataka
16.	Veterinary College	**Bangalore**	Karnataka
17.	Veterinary College	**Hassan**	Karnataka
18.	Veterinary College	**Shimoga**	Karnataka
19.	College of Veterinary and Animal Sciences	**Trichur**	Kerala
20.	College of Veterinary and Animal Sciences	**Pookot**	Kerala
21.	College of Veterinary Science and Animal Husbandry	**Jabalpur**	Madhya Pradesh
22.	College of Veterinary Science and Animal Husbandry	**Mhow**	Madhya Pradesh
23.	College of Veterinary Science and Animal Husbandry	**Rewa**	Madhya Pradesh
24.	College of Veterinary Science and Animal Science	**Parbhani**	Maharashtra
25.	Bombay Veterinary College	**Mumbai**	Maharashtra
26.	Nagapur Veterinary College	**Nagapur**	Maharashtra
27.	K.N.P. College of Veterinary Sciences	**Shirwal**	Maharashtra
28.	Post Graduate Institute of Veterinary and Animal Sciences	**Akola**	Maharashtra
29.	College of Veterinary and Animal Sciences	**Udgir**	Maharashtra
30.	College of Veterinary Science and Animal Husbandry	**Aizawal**	Manipur
31.	College of Veterinary Science and Animal Husbandry	**Bhubaneswar**	Orissa

Contd...

Table–*Contd...*

Sl.No.	*Name of the Colleges*		*State*
32.	Rajeev Gandhi College of Veterinary and Animal Sciences	**Pondicherry**	Pondicherry
33.	College of Veterinary Science	**Ludhiana**	Punjab
34.	College of Veterinary and Animal Science	**Bikaner**	Rajasthan
35.	Apollo College of Veterinary Medicine	**Jaipur**	Rajasthan
36.	Mahatma Gandhi College of Veterinary Science	**Bharatpur**	Rajasthan
37.	Madras Veterinary College	**Chennai**	Tamil Nadu
38.	Veterinary College and Research Institute	**Namakkal**	Tamil Nadu
39.	College of Veterinary Science and Animal Husbandry	Mathura	Uttar Pradesh
40.	College of Veterinary Science and Animal Husbandry	**Faizabad**	Uttar Pradesh
41.	Indian Veterinary Research Institute, Izatnagar	**Barrielly**	Uttar Pradesh
42.	College of Veterinary and Animal Sciences	**Pantnagar**	Uttaranchal
43.	College of Veterinary Science and Animal Sciences	**Kolkatta**	West Bengal

The main goals and objectives of the Veterinary Colleges are:

- ☆ To impart education in different branches of veterinary and animal sciences.
- ☆ To produce competent and skilled veterinary graduates.
- ☆ To provide for applied and fundamental need based research in the field of veterinary and animal sciences.
- ☆ To update the knowledge of farmers regarding the latest technologies in animal health and production.
- ☆ To provide a linkage between the livestock farmers and the concerned industries so as to provide better marketing facilities to the livestock products.
- ☆ To provide a continuous education to the field veterinarians, researchers and extension workers in the field of veterinary and animal sciences.

4.3 Trends in Veterinary Education

Job Orientation Programmes

There is a need to reorient veterinary curricula and syllabi to satisfy the needs of the livestock and poultry industries. The aptitude as well as the skill of veterinarians needs to be improved. It should envision a society in the future in which more veterinarians will opt for private practice rather than government jobs. Already the impact of privatization is being felt in metropolitan cities, where there is a huge private practice sector, especially for companion animals.

Continuing Veterinary Education for Academic Staff Development

Continuing Veterinary Education (CVE) is gaining momentum slowly in the developing countries, including the Indian subcontinent. When properly conducted, CVE is an effective tool to maintain professional competence. To keep pace with the information explosion, veterinary graduates must be informed of the latest developments in the field of veterinary science so that they can effectively deliver the goods.

University–Industry Link

Educational institutions must have continual interaction with industries, institutions, and organizations. The universities must review their academic programmes and reorient the syllabus content to meet the needs of their society.

New Programs

New educational programmes must be launched to serve the dairy, meat, poultry, and fisheries industries. This will help entrepreneurs to invest in those industries. The Tamil Nadu Veterinary and Animal Science University at Chennai, the torchbearer in veterinary education in India, has restructured its curriculum and syllabi, both undergraduate and post-graduate, to suit these needs and plans to offer, or has already launched, the following new educational programs;

- Post-graduate diploma in Animal Business Management.
- MBA in Animal Business Management.
- Veterinary Nursing.

- ☆ Veterinary Pharmaceutics and Drug Delivery System.
- ☆ Entrepreneurship development program on Dairy and meat products.
- ☆ Post-graduate courses in Fish Diseases.
- ☆ Post-graduate courses in Animal Biotechnology.
- ☆ Post-graduate courses in Wild Animal Management.
- ☆ Molecular Biology.
- ☆ Post-graduate diploma in Poultry Diseases.

Integrating models of curricula with those for research and extension in veterinary education is the need of hour in order to keep pace with modern technology. The only way that rural development can be brought out is by launching people centered development programs. A subsistence farmer learns to be a commercial producer; a change necessitates new experiences, new propositions, and practical knowledge. A university that concentrates on helping people to discover new ways of being and on encouraging them to find new ways of learning and doing is much more likely to contribute to sustainable, equitable, and environmentally responsible development than conventional institutions (Rahman, 2004).

4.4 Veterinary Library Systems: Networks and Consortium

Body of a healthy living organism is the best example of life most effective and successful information system. Any change in its atmosphere inside its body systems is immediately informed to the concerned unit and reactions to the change take place instantly. Its reaction is based on the database stored in its memory or function assigned to the particular organ *e.g.* entry of antigen prompts the formation of antibody; similarly a pinprick will result in opposite movement of that body part. An intact information system makes a living body alive or functioning. Similar is the situation with man-made systems - right information at right time is crucial for the existence of any system. Intensive management of animal has changed their world. Latest information on any aspect of animal management may change the situation of animals in a given place.

4.4.1 Information Systems and Network

The information system requires source of information or origin of message, a transmitter who transmits the information throughout a medium, and users. For promoting application of science to matters of collective importance, *viz.*, animals, fishes, animal genetic resources, so-called mission - oriented agencies, national or international, have developed information system of their own that cut across conventional frontiers between disciplines. Many of these systems have been set up by agencies under the United Nations (UN). For instance Agricultural Research Information System (AGRIS) administered by Food and Agriculture Organization (FAO) in India, Medical Literature Analysis and Retrieval System (MEDLARS) of the National Library of Medicine (USA), CAB International (UK) etc.

Realizing the importance of information and data support only in area of national development, international inter-governmental organizations have provided technical assistance to developing countries to improve their national information infrastructures and to benefit from information flow and exchange among themselves and between them and developed countries. In this connection, international co-operative information systems and programmes have facilitated the introduction of programmes and activities at international level, leading to formation of international information systems. For example, CAB international, UK; Institute of Scientific Organization, Philadelphia, USA; Food and Agriculture Organization, Rome; Asia Pacific Centre of Technology Transfer. CGIAR Centers, USA; etc. arc working as international information systems.

Information systems are Libraries and Information Centers, Documentation Centers, Information Analysis Centers, Data Centers, Information Clearing Houses, Depositories, Reprographic Centers, Archives, Extension Centers etc., that strive to support the academic and research needs of veterinary sciences and allied subjects with print and online information resources. These libraries build up a balanced collection chiefly of interest to parent organizations, render personalized services, and provide advanced services to the users. Advanced libraries provide translation service, SDI service, compilation of bibliographies locating information and maintenance of indexed file of selected topics.

An organization which selects acquires stores and retrieves specific documents in response to requests, announces abstracts, extracts and index documents: and disseminate documents in response to request for documents or for contents is called Information / Documentation centre. These are available at International / Regional/ National and Local level. Their important activities include management and administrative services, internal operating services, and external user services. The main services of an information centre are answer the technical queries, literature searches, current awareness services, translation services and preparation of bibliographies. For instance these centers are located at G B Paul University of Agriculture and Technology (Pantnagar). Central Institute of Research on Goat (Makhdoom, Mathura), National Bureau of Animal Genetic Resources (Karnal), Central Marine Fisheries Research Institute (Cochin), National Bureau of Fish Genetic Resources (Lucknow) etc.

An organization where indexing, abstracting, translating, synthesizes and evaluation of information or data in a given field or for a specific mission to provide a definite user group with digested, repacked information or data is called Information Analysis Centers (IAC) ARIC in (ICAR. Delhi). INSDOC now called as NISCAIR (CSIR. Delhi), Agricultural Information Centre, IARI (Delhi) etc. It prepares products after analysis of information and consolidation in the form of state-of-the art reports, reviews, critical reviews, handbooks, trend reports, manuals. Any organization, which meets the potential needs of the users for data obtained from various sources, is called Data Centre. This compiles, evaluates and disseminates data and offers data services. For instance recently ICAR has launched Data Bank at CIRG (Makhdoom), NBAGR (Karnal). IVRI (Izatnagar). Veterinary Service Data Bank. USA, Veterinary Medicine Data Program (USA), etc.

4.4.2 Information Resource Sharing and Consortia

The National Policy on Library and Information System (1988) had recommended use of information technology on a national level. Under Agricultural Research Information System (ARIS), ICAR has given main thrust on Information System Development (ISD), networking and creating infrastructure at headquarters, its institutes, central state-agricultural universities for inter-connectivity with all national, international animal Veterinary/Fishery/Agricultural research institutes and central/Deemed/State Agricultural Universities through e-mail and Internet.

Agricultural research, the backbone of agricultural growth in the country, demands timely dissemination of knowledge being generated and updated across the globe from time to time. With the advent of internet facilities and advancement of web technology, almost all reputed international journals are available on-line and can easily be accessed by researchers over the network. Since ICAR is having network connectivity across the institutes and state agricultural universities, select journals could be made available over the network for the use of scientific community. Keeping this broad objective in mind, the NAIP has established the Consortium for e-Resources in Agriculture (CeRA) at the Indian Agricultural Research Institute (IARI). The NAIP is to facilitate accelerated and sustainable transformation of Indian agriculture in support of poverty alleviation and income generation by collaborative development and application of agricultural innovation by the public research organizations in partnership with the farmer's groups, the private sector, the civil society organizations and other stakeholders.

The objectives of the CeRA are:

- ☆ To develop the existing R and D information resource base of ICAR institutes/universities, etc., comparable to that existing in world leading institutions/organizations.
- ☆ To create an e-access culture among scientists/teachers in ICAR institutes/agricultural universities.
- ☆ To develop a Science Citation Index (SCI) Facility at IARI for evaluation of scientific publications.
- ☆ To assess the impact of CeRA on the level of research publications measured through SCI.

4.4.3 Campus Network of Veterinary College Library

India, being an agrarian country, the growth of agriculture is reflected in the good yields of different crops that depend on various factors – natural and man-made. Agricultural research, the backbone of agricultural growth in the country, demands timely dissemination of knowledge that is generated and updated across the globe from time-to-time. India is fast emerging as a preferred destination for agriculture education, especially at post graduate and doctoral level.

India is known world over for the quality of teaching, training and research in agriculture and allied sciences as also quality education in animal sciences, dairy and fishery sectors.

Library, which forms the integral part and a great source of information for animal sciences, dairy and fishery sectors, constitutes heart of the Veterinary College by organizing, processing and providing access to information to its users at right time in convenient format. Under the present scenario, most of the libraries in the world are plagued by shortage of funds. Due to ever increasing cost of published material, the library collections are shrinking. In contrast to this, the user demands are increasing. Libraries are at their wits' end to satisfy the needs of their clientele. The only viable solution to meet user's demand is to make optimum use of available literature. This is being done through pooling and sharing of resources like print as well as electronics by way of consortia. The primary mission of an organization's ICT operation is to ensure the cost-effective delivery of ICT services that allow the organization to achieve its mandate. To meet this objective, the organization must determine the most efficient manner to deliver services; i.e., whether to host certain ICT services internally or externally. Clearly, this decision has an impact on both the quality benefits and the costs of the service delivered.

With the advent of Internet facilities and advancement of web technology, almost all reputed international journals are available on-line and can easily be accessed by researchers over the network. Since ICAR is having network connectivity across the institutes and state agricultural universities, select journals could be made available over the network for the use of scientific community. Keeping this broad objective in mind, the National Agricultural Innovative Programme (NAIP) has established the Consortium for e-Resources in Agriculture (CeRA) at the Indian Agricultural Research Institute (IARI) to develop the existing R and D information resources of ICAR institutes/universities providing online access to major e-publishers viz., Springer (890 journals), Annual reviews (22 journals) and CSIRO (8 journals). To achieve resource sharing among veterinary college libraries for effective information management, provide access and communication to support learning, teaching, research and extension activities. A strong State-of-the-Art ICT facilities and network base is very much essential in every Veterinary College of India by establishing Campus Network. This will definitely boost the collections of the Veterinary libraries and will also cater to the information needs of undergraduates, postgraduates, scientists and faculty members engaged in education, research and extension activities of veterinary colleges in India.

An attempt has been made in the following paragraphs to provide guidelines to the authorities, which includes Computer Managers and Library professionals in establishing the Local Area Network (LAN) and a National/ International Network (WAN) at Veterinary Colleges in India, with a motto to optimize the e-resources on the Internet; share and exchange information resources and build strong communication bond among peer groups sitting at their desktops around the clock by overcoming regional barriers.

Taking into consideration of the existing situation of network facilities and consortium facilities available and accessed in the Veterinary College Libraries in India, the first and foremost requirement is to have sound Information and Communication Technology infrastructure among each and every Veterinary College Library in India. Figure 4.1 depicts the Campus Network of Veterinary College for building a planned network foundation, a must to access Internet and e-resources to a large extent by all the students and teaching faculty in Veterinary and allied sciences.

Figure 4.1 depicts the proposed campus network of Veterinary College, which needs to be established in every college for networking and resource sharing and this in turn leads to national network. The campus network should be connected to campus clinical blocks, Departments, Digital Library, Administrative blocks and Hostels by drawing Fiber optics using dedicated leased line which may range from 2 mbps to 10 mbps. Each block should have a terminated data switch for extra connectivity of nodes and CAT 6 cable may be used within the unit/ block. It is clear from the figure that, all the blocks of a veterinary college are connected to a data switch in turn to router for network connectivity. This will ensure smooth flow of data, effective communication, database management, e-governance and thereby contribute for establishing national networks.

Budget Estimate for Establishing Network Facilities in a Veterinary College is shown in Table 4.1, which provides a clear picture about the technical infrastructure and allied components required for campus network in a Veterinary Colleges.

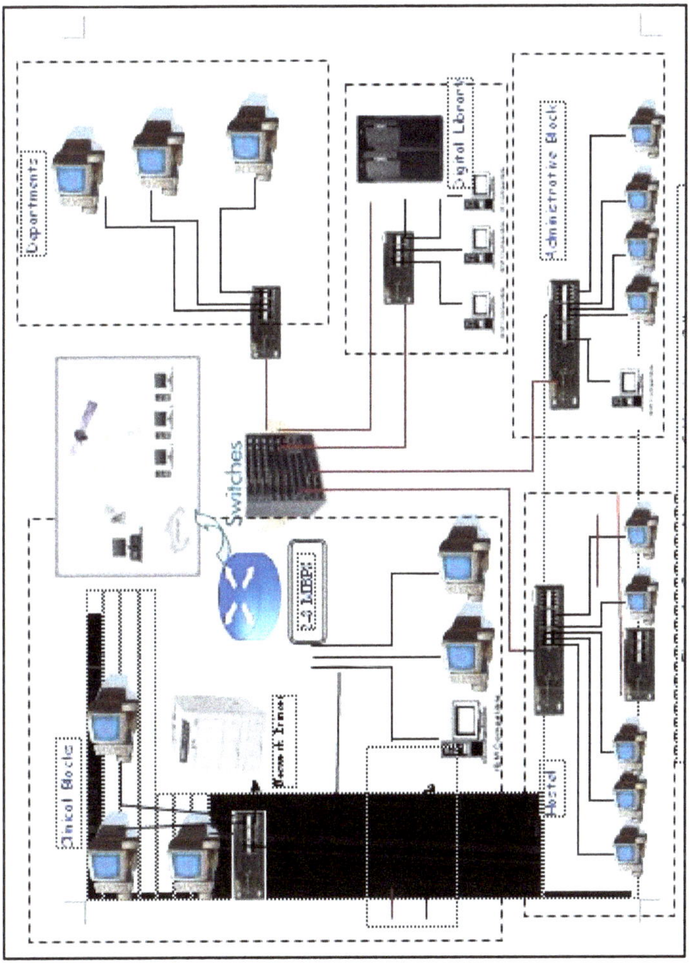

Figure 4.1: Campus Network of Veterinary College

Table 4.1: Budget Estimate for Establishing Network Facilities in a Veterinary College

Equipments	*Configuration (Minimum)*	*Students*		*Departments and Clinical Blocks*	*Quantity*	*Cost (in lakhs)*
		UG (300) (1:10)	*PG and PhD (100) (1:5)*	*(20) (1:5)*		
Computer Systems	Pentium IV	30	20	100	150	45.00
Main Servers	Quad Core Intel® Xeon® E% 310, Cache Server, Hot Swap, Raid Controller	–	–	–	2	9.00
OFC Cable and E-CAT Cable	Single and Double core, CAT 6 or higher	–	–	–	2 bundles (based on plinth area)	4.00
Data Optic Switches	CISCO or D-Link (24 port and higher)	–	–	–		1.50
Firewall	Anti-virus (Corporate edition)	–	–	–		0.90
Internet Bandwidth	Leased Line (Min. 2 mbps)	–	–	–		3.70
Manpower for network setup	Technical Personnel	–	–	–		1.00
Total		–	–	–		**65.10**
Annual Maintenance Contract	Reserve 10% of the total cost of equipments	–	–	–		5.00

The strength of students on an average enrolled in the Veterinary Colleges in India are between 300 and 400 students comprising of undergraduates, postgraduates and Research scholars based on the results of Table 4.1.

Each Veterinary College needs to set up campus network by initial investment of Rs 65.10 lakh, which may vary from one institute to other in the interest of effective information transfer and e-governance. Although the approximated cost (vide Table 1) looks bit high, it should be noted that it is an one time investment for long term benefit.

4.4.4 Establishing Veterinary Library Network (VETLIBNET)

VETLIBNET (Veterinary Library Network) is a proposed network of libraries (Figure 4.2) under the purview of Veterinary Council of India covering 44 Veterinary Colleges in India, whose main mission is to create a virtual network of Library information sources and services to provide effective and efficient access to knowledge through perseverance, innovation and collaboration. In this direction, Indian Veterinary Research Institute (IVRI), being one of the premier research institutions with deemed university status can take lead in establishing Library network for all the Veterinary institutes in the country. By establishing campus network in all the Veterinary College Libraries as proposed earlier, cost on establishing Veterinary Library Network at national level would be easier. By establishing national network, individual libraries will be benefited by the resources available in the veterinary libraries at national level.

The major activities and functions of this proposed VETLIBNET (Veterinary Library Network) are to strive to devise and execute the following:

Database management should be of high priority insisting on library automation in each and every Veterinary College Library and thereby creating databases of books, Serials Holdings, Current Serials, Theses, Experts and Research Projects. To achieve this, national policy be framed in selecting a uniform library software for consistency and compatibility so that union catalogue of participating libraries can be established acting as a national gateway to the veterinary information resources to the world at large.

Developing standards and uniform guidelines in techniques, methods, procedures, computer hardware and software, services

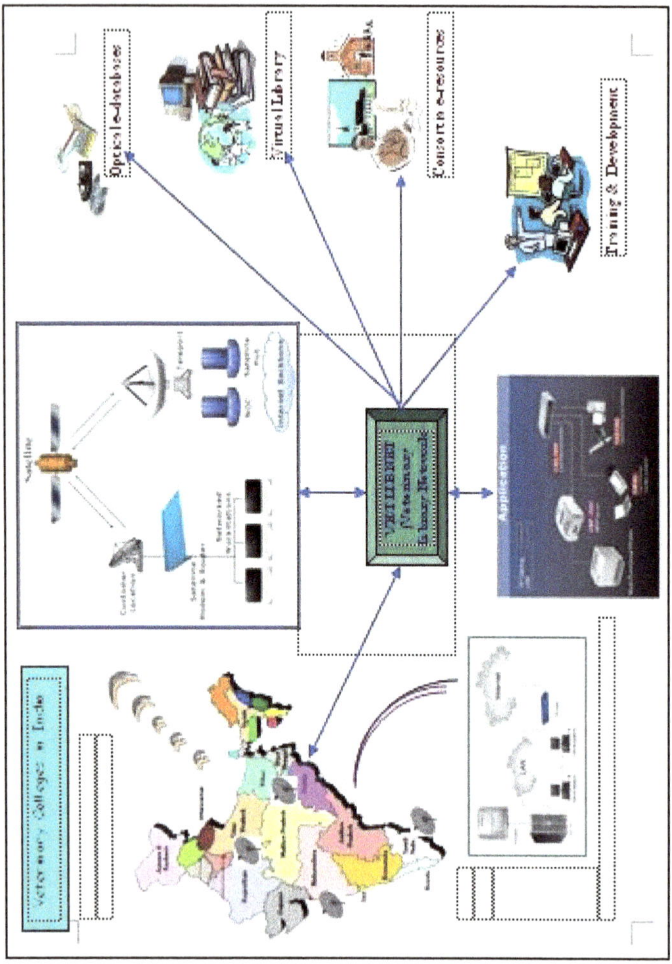

Figure 4.2: Proposed Model for Networking of Veterinary College Libraries in India

and promote their adoption in actual practice by all libraries, in order to facilitate pooling, sharing and exchange of information towards optimal use of resources and facilities.

The databases of all individual libraries will be merged. This has a major advantage from the user's point of view; it will be easy to veterinarians as well as faculty and students to access /get required information where the centralized databases are available. The unique library software is very much essential for creating the database and accessing the information from central node.

National consortium exclusively in the field of Veterinary Sciences should be worked out to identify core journals and databases of relevance to support academic and research activities of Veterinarians/ scientists in the country.

Manpower Resources

To build and strengthen ICT infrastructure in every Veterinary College Library by providing financial, technical and ICT infrastructure with the help of Indian Council of Agricultural Research (ICAR), drawing intellectual manpower plays significant role, as they are involved in rendering information services to the users. At this juncture, status of the library professional plays an important role in drawing intellectuals to the profession. The Librarians should be provided with status, attractive monetary benefits.

This call for better status and importance is given in recruiting required staff in the veterinary college libraries for effectively serving the users. Under these circumstances, unless library staffs are given status and due benefit establishing proposed ICT infrastructure and ICT based services would not be possible. As such, regular education and training should be imparted to the library professionals working across the country so that the emerging technologies could be properly implemented in their respective libraries. Further national meets/ conferences be organized every year as a platform for exchange of ideas/ skills and keeping up-to-date in the development of the library and information science.

References and Further Readings

Arvindan M. (2002). Animal Science Education in India. *Handbook of Animal Husbandry*: ICAR, New Delhi, pp.1033-1041.

Consortium for e-Resources in Agriculture. available at www.cera.jccc.in (Accessed on 14th July, 2009).

ICAR Report (2004). Conference of State Ministers of Animal husbandry and Dairy Development in 11th Dec., 2004 in National Agricultural Science Complex, Pusa, New Delhi. Pp. 1 - 17.

Jogi, S. (2004). VCI Regulations: A boon or bane of veterinary education. *Pashudhan*,. 30 (04): 5.

Livestock census of India (2003). Available at www.livestock census, (Accessed on 28th April, 2009).

Kumar Aruna T, (2002.) Informatics in Animal Husbandry. Handbook of Animal Husbandry. New Delhi: ICAR, pp.1168-1187.

Pawar Sachin, S. Saravanan and Suhas Amrutkar, (2009). Biotechnology: A tool for Dairy Development in India. *Dairy Planner*, 5 (05): 20-21.

Rahman S Abdul (2004). The History of Veterinary Education in India. *Journal of Veterinary Medical Education*, 31 (1):55-60.

Singh Jasvinder and Verma Harish Kumar (2007). A peep in to Veterinary Profession. *Pashudhan*, 33(8): 1-4.

Veterinary Council of India. Available at www.vci.nic.in (Accessed on 14th July, 2009).

Chapter 5

Literature Survey and Citation Manuals

5.1 Concept of Literature Survey

Literature survey is background work that is made in groups as a part of the assignment. It is based on books, scientific journals, indexing and abstracting databases and academic publications. The main goal of a literature survey is to gather a basis for the practical work and to show that the student is familiar with existing literature and research on the topic. It is crucial to be familiar with the field, *i.e.* the concepts, methods and their applications, in order to apply them correctly in one's own assignment or research work.

Literature survey is the documentation of a comprehensive review of the published and unpublished work from secondary sources data in the areas of specific interest to the researcher. The library is a rich storage base for secondary data and researchers used to spend several weeks and sometimes months going through books, journals, newspapers, magazines, conference proceedings, doctoral dissertations, master's theses, government publications and financial reports to find information on their research topic. With computerized databases now readily available and accessible the literature search is much speedier and easier and can be done without entering the portals of a library building.

The researcher could start the literature survey even as the information from the unstructured and structured interviews is being gathered. Reviewing the literature on the topic area at this time helps the researcher to focus further interviews more meaningfully on certain aspects found to be important is the published studies even if these had not surfaced during the earlier questioning. So the literature survey is important for gathering the secondary data for the research which might be proved very helpful in the research. The literature survey can be conducted for several reasons. The literature review can be in any area of the field.

Literature survey is undertaken in the process of choosing/ identifying a new problem of research, compiling information on a particular topic, in depth understanding of concept, know the development and trend of a subject or sub-subject etc literature survey call for literature review.

A literature review discusses published information in a particular subject area, and sometimes information in a particular subject area within a certain time period. A literature review can be just a simple summary of the sources, but it usually has an organizational pattern and combines both summary and synthesis. A summary is a recap of the important information of the source, but a synthesis is a re-organization, or a reshuffling, of that information. It might give a new interpretation of old material or combine new with old interpretations or it might trace the intellectual progression of the field.

According to Cooper (1988)

"... a literature review uses as its database reports of primary or original scholarship, and does not report new primary scholarship itself. The primary reports used in the literature may be verbal, but in the vast majority of cases reports are written documents. The types of scholarship may be empirical, theoretical, critical/analytic, or methodological in nature. Second a literature review seeks to describe summaries, evaluate, clarify and/or integrate the content of primary reports."

A literature review may constitute an essential chapter of a thesis or dissertation in academic university setup for the award of degree either masters or Post Graduation or PhD. The main purpose of literature reviews is to:

- Insight the status of development of concept.
- Show the research work in the context of its contribution to the understanding of the subject under review.
- Establish the relationship of each work to the others under consideration.
- Resolve conflicts amongst seemingly contradictory previous studies.
- Identify areas of prior scholarship to prevent duplication of effort.
- Points out the way for future areas of research and serve as a guideline for the upcoming research community.
- Substantiate the authors for contributing the research work.

5.2 Steps in Literature Survey

A literature review will generally be part of a thesis or dissertation, forming an early context-setting chapter. It may also form a useful background for outlining a piece of research, or putting forward a hypothesis. The steps involved in conducting literature review are

Define the Research Problem

Understand the research problem in question and identify the concepts or components of research title or problem based on the objectives of the study.

Identify the Relevant Library Sources

The information sources that are relevant for writing literature review on the research problem are mainly secondary sources in addition to the following sources *i.e.:*

- Books (monographs, textbooks, reference books).
- Research articles from journals.
- Newspaper articles.
- Indexing and abstracting databases.
- Technical and government reports and statistical information.
- Theses and dissertations etc.

Secondary sources are first step to be consulted for conducting literature review and some of them in the field of agriculture and veterinary databases are:

- Veterinary Science Abstracts
- JCCC@CeRA
- Biological Abstracts
- Agricola
- Food Science and Technology Abstracts

5.3 Evaluate the Usefulness of Library Sources

It is essential to evaluate the authority and worthiness of the document reviewed. More specifically, author's credentials, date of publication peer reviewed journal etc. needs to be considered. The evaluation of appraisal based on content analysis for literature review should ensure the following:

- Is the writer addressing a scholarly audience?
- Does the author review the relevant literature?
- Does the author write from an objective viewpoint, and are their views based on facts rather than opinions?
- Does the design sound?
- Is it primary or secondary material?
- Does the author have a particular theoretical viewpoint?
- What is the relationship of this work to other material?
- Is the author's argument logically organized and clear to follow?

Analyze the Findings

Literature review should discus the findings and conclusions of pertinent literature and should be reported accordingly.

- Structure of a literature survey
- Title and author
- Name, student id and other information as usual
- Abstract (summary)
- Brief presentation of the content

- Keywords
- Give a list of names of essential concepts, approaches and methods that you have covered in your work
- Do not just collect some words that just sound nice
- Introduction
- What is the topic and why it is important
- To what larger wholeness the survey topic belongs
- What you plan to accomplish in your literature survey
- Body: this is where you discuss your sources. Here are some ways in which you could organize your discussion:

Chronologically

For example, if writers' views have tended to change over time. There is little point in doing the review by order of publication unless this shows a clear trend.

Thematically

Take particular themes in the literature, for example in the literature review of poverty and disability cited in the next section, the author takes the themes of the prevalence and structure of disability, education, employment, income and poverty, causes of disability, the path from poverty to disability and vice versa, and finally, policies for disabled people.

Methodologically

The focus is on the methods of the researcher, for example, qualitative versus quantitative approaches.

Conclusions

Summarize the major contributions, evaluating the current position, and pointing out flaws in methodology, gaps in the research, contradictions, and areas for further study.

References

- A good list of reference is important
- Has to follow some known referencing practice (*e.g.* Harvard referencing)

5.4 Bibliography/Citation Skills

A bibliography is usually thought of as an alphabetical listing of books at the end of a written work either book, book chapter, or article, to which the author referred during the research and writing process. In addition to books, bibliographies can include sources such as articles, reports, interviews, or even non-print resources like Web sites, video or audio recordings. Because they may include such varied resources, bibliographies are also referred to as 'references', 'works cited' or 'works consulted' the latter can include those titles that merely contributed to research, but were not specifically cited in text.

Dr S.R. Ranganathan defines bibliography as a "list of documents together for some purpose and is to bring to the attention of the reader an exhaustive or selective list of documents relevant to his/ her pursuit of study or enquiry".

The standard bibliography details the citation information of the consulted sources: author(s), date of publication, title, and publisher's name and location (and for articles: journal title, volume, issue and page numbers). The primary function of bibliographic citations is to assist the reader in finding the sources used in the writing of a work. To these basic citations, the annotated bibliography adds descriptive and evaluative comments (i.e., an annotation), assessing the nature and value of the cited works. The addition of commentary provides the future reader or researcher essential critical information and a foundation for further research.

The UNESCO and the Library of Congress in their survey of bibliographical services, conducted in 1950, have stated the following aims and functions of bibliography:

- Its aim is to make it possible for intellectual workers, to learn of publications recording the developments in their fields of interest not only in their own countries but also through the world.
- Promote the effectiveness of a particular project in research.
- Contribute to the cultural development and enjoyment which are derived from records of learning and culture.
- Assist in promoting useful applications of existing knowledge and in making the applications which have been developed in one country, widely known to all countries.

Ex:

- ☆ British National Bibliography, London: Council of the British National Bibliography; London: British Library Bibliographies Services Division.
- ☆ Indian National Bibliography, Calcutta: Central Reference Library, National Library.

Preparation of Bibliography

Bibliographic references and citations are crucial to academic work because they are the means by which authors acknowledge and identify the sources of their ideas and information. For any research paper or book, writing a bibliography is essential, to prevent any accusations of plagiarism, and to give fair credit to the work of previous authors in the field.

In order to prepare and compile bibliography various citation manuals are available which needs to be adhered to compile a bibliography. Here the term citations refer to the references cited in the book or article for writing or publishing a journal article or book. Citation is a reference to a published or unpublished source like reference to a book, article, web page, or other published item. The objective of a citation is to acknowledge the intellectual honesty of the sources used or consulted.

During compilation of bibliographies or citations, there are different manuals which are practiced. Among them, the important citation manuals are:

1. Harvard System (http://libweb.anglia.ac.uk/referencing/harvard.htm)
2. Modern Language Association (MLA) Style (http://honolulu.hawaii.edu/library/mlahcc.html)
3. American Psychological Association (http://en.wikipedia.org/wiki/APA_style)

5.4.1 HARVARD SYSTEM (http://libweb.anglia.ac.uk/referencing/harvard.htm)

During the course of writing an essay, report or other assignment it is usual to support arguments by reference to other published work. These references may be from work presented in journal or newspaper articles, government reports, books or specific chapters of books, research dissertations or theses, material over the internet etc. Citation is the practice of referring to the work of other authors in the text of your own piece of work. Such works are cited to show evidence both of the background reading that has been done and to support the content and conclusions. Each citation requires a reference at the end of the work; this gives the full details of the source item and should enable it to be traced. Referring accurately to such source materials is part of sound academic practice and a skill that should be mastered. Other reasons for accurate citation and referencing are:

- To give credit to the concepts and ideas of other authors.
- To provide the reader (often the marker/examiner of the assignment) with evidence of the breadth and depth of your reading.
- To enable those who read your work to locate the cited references easily Remember to note the details of all the documents you read. The following pages give detailed guidance for various types of documents as there are major differences between books, journal articles and websites. These are based on consultation with colleagues at Anglia Ruskin University, with examples, in red, for illustrative purposes.

When citing published works, the Harvard system should be used. In this system, the author's name and the year of publication should be given in the text in one of the following forms:

CITING REFERENCES IN TEXT

Author's Name Cited in the Text

When making reference to an author's work in your text, their name is followed by the year of publication of their work:

> In general, when writing for a professional publication, it is good practice to make reference to other relevant published work. This view has been supported in the work of Cormack (1994).

Where you are mentioning a particular part of the work, and making direct reference to this, a page reference should be included:

> Cormack (1994, pp.32-33) states that 'when writing for a professional readership, writers invariably make reference to already published works'.

Author's Name Not Cited Directly in the Text

If you make reference to a work or piece of research without mentioning the author in the text then both the author's name and publication year are placed at the relevant point in the sentence or at the end of the sentence in brackets:

> Making reference to published work appears to be characteristic of writing for a professional audience (Cormack, 1994).

More than One Author Cited in the Text

Where reference is made to more than one author in a sentence, and they are referred to directly, they are both cited:

> Jones (1946) and Smith (1948) have both shown ...

More than One Author Not Cited Directly in the Text

List these at the relevant point in the sentence or at the end of the sentence, putting the author's name, followed by the date of publication and separated by a semi-colon and within brackets:

> Where several publications from a number of authors are referred to, then the references should be cited in chronological order (*i.e.* earliest first):

Further research in the late forties (Jones, 1946; Smith, 1948) lead to major developments......

(Collins, 1998; Brown, 2001; Davies, 2008)

Two, Three or Four Authors for the Same Work

When there are two authors for a work they should both be noted in the text:

> White and Brown (2004) in their recent research paper found...with regard to PREP and the role of libraries, Crane and Urquhart (1994) suggest...

or indirectly, using an and:

During the mid nineties research undertaken in Luton (Slater and Jones, 1996) showed that...

or

Earlier research (White and Brown, 1966) demonstrated that the presence of certain chemicals would lead to...

More than Four Authors for a Work

Where there are several authors (more than four), only the first author should be used, followed by **'et al.'** meaning **and others**:

Green, *et al.* (1995) found that the majority ...

or indirectly:

Recent research (Green, *et al.*, 1995) has found that the majority of ...

Several Works by One Author in Different Years

If more than one publication from an author illustrates the same point and the works are published in different years, then the references should be cited in chronological order (*i.e.* earliest first):

as suggested by Bloggs (1992, 1994) who found that ...

or indirectly:

research in the nineties (Bloggs 1992, 1994) found that ...

Several Works by One Author in the Same Year

If you are quoting several works published by the same author in the same year, they should be differentiated by adding a lower case letter directly, with no space, after the year for each item:

Earlier research by Dunn (1993a) found that...but later research suggested again by Dunn (1993b) that ...

If several works published in the same year are referred to on a single occasion, or an author has made the same point in several publications, they can all be referred to by using lower case letters (as above):

Bloggs (1993a, b) has stated on more than one occasion that ...

Chapter Authors in Edited Works

References to the work of an author that appears as a chapter, or part of a larger work, that is edited by someone else, should be cited within your text using the name of the contributory author not the editor of the whole work.

In his work on health information, Smith (1975) states ...

In the reference list at the end of your document, you should include details of both the chapter author and the editor of the entire work.

Corporate Authors

If the work is by a recognised organisation and has no personal author then it is usually cited under the body that commissioned the work. This applies to publications by associations, companies, government departments etc. such as Department of the Environment or Royal College of Nursing.

It is acceptable to use standard abbreviations for these bodies, *e.g.* RCN, in your text, providing that the full name is given at the first citing with the abbreviation in brackets:

1st citation:

... research in 2006 undertaken by the Royal College of Nursing (RCN) has shown that ...

2nd citation:

More recently the RCN (2007) has issued guidelines ...

Note that the full name is the preferred format in the reference list. Some reports are written by specially convened groups or committees and can be cited by the name of the committee:

Committee on Nursing (1972)

Select Committee on Stem Cell Research (2002)

Note there are some exceptions to this such as

BBC Philharmonic Orchestra

BBC News

where the abbreviations or initials form part of the official name.

No Author

If the author cannot be identified use '**Anonymous**' or '**Anon**' and the title of the work and date of publication. The title should be written in italics. Every effort should be made to establish the authorship if you intend to use this work as supporting evidence in an academic submission:

Marketing strategy (Anon., 1999).

No Date

The abbreviation **n.d.** is used to denote this:

Smith (n.d.) has written and demonstrated......

or indirectly:

Earlier research (Smith, n.d.) demonstrated that......

Every effort should be made to establish the year of publication if you intend to use this work as supporting evidence in an academic submission.

Page Numbers

Including the page numbers of a reference will help readers trace your sources. This is particularly important for quotations and for paraphrasing specific paragraphs in the text:

Lawrence (1966, p.124) states "we should expect..."

or indirectly:

This is to be expected (Lawrence 1966, p.124)...

Please note page numbers: preceded with p. for a single page.and pp. for a range of pages.

Quoting Portions of Published Text

If you want to include text from a published work in your essay then the sentence(s) must be included within quotation marks, and may be introduced by such phrases as:

the author states that "........"

or

the author writes that "........"

In order for a reader to trace the quoted section it is good practice to give the number of the page where the quotation was found. The quotation should also be emphasized (especially if it runs to 50 words or more) by indenting it and using quotation marks. This clearly identifies the quotation as the work of someone else:

On the topic of professional writing and referencing Cormack (1994, p.32) states:

'When writing for a professional readership, writers invariably make reference to already published works'.

Secondary Sources (Second-hand references)

You may come across a summary of another author's work in the source you are reading, which you would like to make reference to in your own document; this is called secondary referencing.

A direct reference:

Research recently carried out in the Greater Manchester area by Brown (1966 cited in Bassett, 1986, p.142) found that ...

In this example, Brown is the work, which you wish to refer to, but have not read directly for yourself. Bassett is the secondary source, where you found the summary of Brown's work.

or Indirectly:

(Brown, 1966 cited in Bassett, 1986, p.142)

In the example below White is the primary or original source and Black is the secondary source. It is important to realise that Black may have taken White's ideas forward, and altered their original meaning. If you need to cite a secondary reference it is recommended that, where possible, you read the original source for yourself rather than rely on someone else's interpretation of a work.

White, (1990) as cited in Black (1994), suggests that...

Tables and Diagrams

When reproducing selected data from a diagram or table, or copying the entire table or diagram, a reference must be made to the source.

A reference within the text to a table taken from *e.g.* a book, should include the author and page (Smith, 2005, p.33) to enable the reader to identify the data. If the source of the data is not the author's own, but obtained from another source, it becomes a secondary reference and needs to be cited as such:

(United Nations, 1975 cited in Smith, 2005, p.33)

If the table is reproduced in its entirety place the citation as a footnote. Be particularly careful to note the original source of data, as well as the authorship of the document. Full details should be included in the reference list.

In the following example, a table is reproduced from page 267, of a book written by Robert Amazon which is the 4th edition and published by FT Prentice Hall of Harlow, England in 2005. The title of the book is Management in the media: decision makers.

- ☆ If you wish to reproduce the table in your own work – replicate the table

Television ownership in England
Percentage of Household

Date	1970	1980
Percentage	60	70

Source: National Statistics Office, 1985 *

and add a Footnote – at the bottom of the page in your own work acknowledging the source of the reproduced table.

- ☆ National Statistics Office 1985 cited in Amazon, 2005, p.267
- ☆ If you wish to quote from a table in the above book in your essay:

  ……..historical figures demonstrate that only sixty percent of households had televisions in Britain by the 1970s (National Statistics Office 1985 cited in Amazon, 2005, p. 267).

- ☆ Ensure you include the book in the reference list or bibliography at the end of your work:

Amazon, R., 2005. *Management in the media: decision makers.* 4th ed. Harlow: FT Prentice Hall.

Websites

When citing material found on a website, you should identify the authorship of the website. This may be a corporate author, an organisation or a company; a guide to this can be found by looking at the URL or web address. To find the date of publication, reference to this might be found at the bottom of a web page relating to copyright, or from a date headline.

In this example the authorship would be BBC and the date 2009.

Recent research on meningitis (BBC, 2009) has shown …

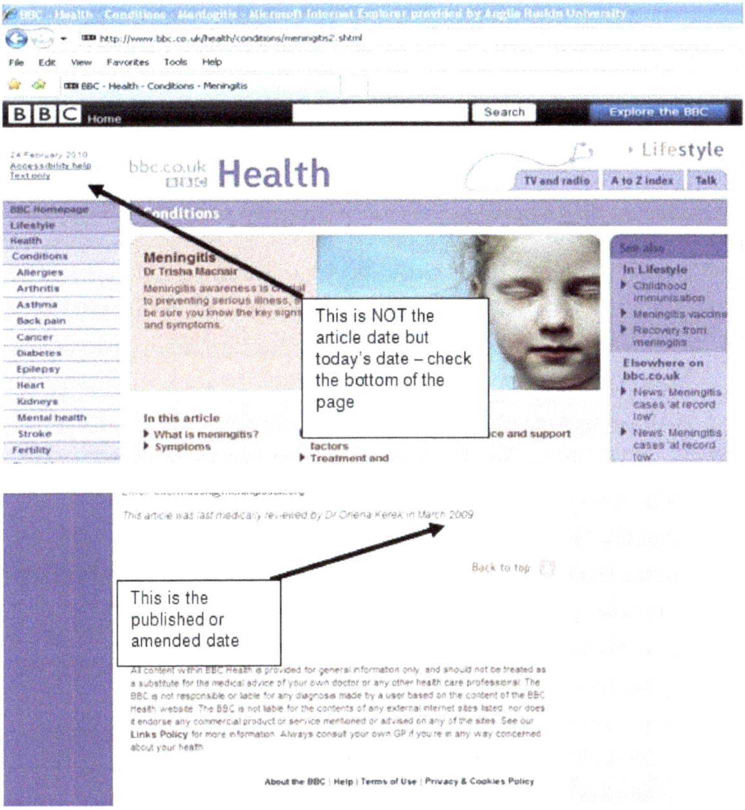

COMPILING THE REFERENCE LIST AND BIBLIOGRAPHY

General Guidelines, Layout and Punctuation

The purpose of a reference list is to enable sources to be easily traced by another reader. Different types of publication require different amounts of information but there are certain common elements such as authorship, year of publication and title.

Section 7 deals with references where some of the details are unknown.

The Harvard style lays down standards for the order and content of information in the reference. Some variations of layout are acceptable provided that they are used consistently.

All items should be listed alphabetically by author or authorship, regardless of the format, *i.e.* whether books, websites or journal articles etc. Where there are several works from one author or source they should by listed together but in date order, with the earliest work listed first.

Books

Books with One Author

Use the title page, not the book cover, for the reference details. Only include the edition where it is not the first. A book with no edition statement is most commonly a first edition.

The required elements for a book reference are:

Author, Initials., Year. *Title of book.* Edition. (only include this if not the first edition) Place of publication (this must be a town or city, not a country): Publisher.

Reference where 1st edition

Baron, D. P., 2008. *Business and the organisation.* Chester: Pearson.

where, 3rd edition

Redman, P., 2006. *Good essay writing: a social sciences guide.* 3rd ed. London: Open University in assoc. with Sage.

An intext reference for the above examples would read:

Organisations have been found to differ (Baron, 2008) when there is ...

Leading social scientists such as Redman (2006) have noted ...

Please note where there is likely to be confusion with UK place names; for USA towns include the State in abbreviated form e.g. Birmingham, AL.

Books with Two, Three or Four Authors

For books with two, three or four authors of equal status the names should all be included in the order they appear in the document. Use to link the last two multiple authors.

The required elements for a reference are: Author, Initials, Year. *Title of book.* Edition (only include this if not the first edition). Place: Publisher.

Reference

Barker, R. Kirk, J. and Munday, R.J., 1988. *Narrative analysis.* 3rd ed. Bloomington: Indiana University Press.

An intext reference for the above examples would read

A new theory (Barker, Kirk and Munday, 1988) has challenged traditional thinking ...

Books with More Than Four Authors

For books where there are more than four authors use the first author only with surname and initials followed by ***et al.***

The required elements for a reference are:

Author, Initials **and** *et al.*, Year. Title of book. Edition (only include this if not the first edition). Place: Publisher.

Reference

Grace, B. *et al.*, 1988. *A history of the world.* Princeton, NJ: Princeton University Press.

Books which are Edited

For books which are edited give the editor(s) surname(s) and initials, followed by **ed.,** or **eds.**

The required elements for a reference are:

Author, Initials., ed., Year. *Title of book.* Edition. Place: Publisher.

Keene, E. ed., 1988. *Natural language.* Cambridge: University of Cambridge Press.

Silverman, D.F. and Propp, K.K. eds., 1990. *The active interview.* Beverly Hills, CA: Sage.

Allouche, Jose. ed., 2006. *Corporate social resposibility, Volume 1: concepts, accountability and reporting.* Basingstoke: Palgrave Macmillan.

Chapters of edited Nooks

For chapters of edited books the required elements for a reference are:

Chapter author(s) surname(s) and initials. Year of chapter. Title of chapter followed by **In:** Book editor(s) initials and surnames with ed. or eds. after the last name. Year of book. Title of book. Place of publication: Publisher. Chapter number or first and last page numbers followed by full-stop.

Reference

Smith, J., 1975. A source of information. In: W. Jones, ed. 2000. *One hundred and one ways to find information about health.* Oxford: Oxford University Press. Ch. 2.

Samson, C., 1970. Problems of information studies in history. In: S. Stone, ed. *Humanities information research.* Sheffield: CRUS, pp. 44-68.

An intext reference for the above example would read:

(Smith, 1975)

(Samson, 1970)

Multiple Works by the Same Author

Where there are several works by one author and published in the same year they should be differentiated by adding a lower case letter after the date.

For multiple works the required elements for a reference are: Author, Initals., Year. *Title of book.* Place: Publisher.

Soros, G., 1966a. *The road to serfdom.* Chicago: University of Chicago Press.

Soros, G., 1966b. *Beyond the road to serfdom.* Chicago: University of Chicago Press.

Works by the same author should be displayed in chronological order, earliest first (as above).

An intext reference for the above example would read:

(Soros, 1966a)

(Soros, 1966b)

This also applies if there are several authors with the same surname. As an alternative their initials can be included in the citation.

So for example, if you have sources written by George Soros and also by Manuel Soros, you would list them in alphabetic order:

(Soros, G. 1966a)

(Soros, G. 1966b)

(Soros, M. 1966)

Books which have been Translated

For works which have been translated the reference should include details of the translator, the suggested elements for such references being:

Author, Year. *Title of book.* Translated from (language) by (name of translator) Place of publication: Publisher.

Canetti, E., 2001. *The voices of Marrakesh: a record of a visit.* Translated from German by J.A.Underwood. San Francisco: Arion.

For major works of historic significance, the date of the original work may be included along with the date of the translation:

Kant, I., 1785. *Fundamental principles of the metaphysic of morals.*Translated by T.K. Abbott., 1988. New York: Prometheus Books.

E-books

For e-books accessed through a password protected database from the University Library the required elements for a reference are:

Author, Year, *Title of book.* [type of medium] Place of publication: Publisher. Followed by "Available through:" include e-book source/ database, web address or URL [Accessed date].

Fishman, R., 2005. *The rise and fall of suburbia.* [e-book] Chester: Castle Press. Available through: Anglia Ruskin University Library <http://libweb.anglia.ac.uk> [Accessed 5 June 2005].

Carlsen, J. and Charters, S., eds. 2007. *Global wine tourism.* [e-book] Wallingford: CABI Pub. Available through: Anglia Ruskin University Library website <www.libweb.anglia.ac.uk> [Accessed 9 June 2008].

For an e-book freely available over the internet:

The required elements for a reference are:

Authorship, Year, *Title of book.* [type of medium] Place of publication (if known): Publisher. Followed by "Available at:" include web address or URL for the e-book [Accessed date].

The required elements for a reference are: Authorship, Year, *Title of book.* [type of medium] Place of publication: Publisher. Followed by "Available at:" include web address or URL for the actual pdf, where available [Accessed date].

Department of Health, 2008. *Health inequalities: progress and next steps.* [pdf] London: Department of Health. Available at: http://www.dh.gov.uk/en/Publicationsandstatistics/Publications/PublicationsPolicyAndGuidance/DH_085307> [Accessed 9 June 2008].

Bank of England, 2008. *Inflation Report* [pdf] Available at: <http://www.bankofengland.co.uk/publications/inflationreport/ir08nov.pdf> [Accessed 20 April 2009].

An in text reference for the above example would read:

Recent evidence (Bank of England, 2008, pp.32-33) show the trends...

Journal Articles and Newspapers

Journal Articles

For journal articles the required elements for a reference are:

Author, Initials., Year. Title of article. *Full Title of Journal,* Volume number (Issue/Part number), Page numbers.

Boughton, J.M., 2002. The Bretton Woods proposal: an indepth look. *Political Science Quarterly,* 42(6), pp.564-78.

Perry, C., 2001. What health care assistants know about clean hands. *Nursing Times,* 97(22), pp.63-64.

Cox, C., 2002. What health care assistants know about clean hands. *Nursing today,* Spring Issue, pp.647-85.

Journal Articles Available from a Database

For journal articles from an electronic source accessed through a password protected database from the University Library the required elements for a reference are:

Author, Initials., Year. Title of article. *Full Title of Journal,* [type of medium] Volume number (Issue/Part number), Page numbers if availalble. Available through: name of database [Accessed date]

Boughton, J.M., 2002. The Bretton Woods proposal: an in depth look. *Political Science Quarterly* [e-journal] 42 (6) Available through: Blackwell Science Synergy database [Accessed 12 June 2005].

Magazine or Journal Articles Available on the Internet

For an article from a web based magazine or journal, which is freely available over the web, the required elements for a reference are:

Authors, Initials., Year . Title of article, *Full Title of Magazine,* [online]. Available at: web address (quote the exact URL for the article) [Accessed date].

Kipper, D., 2008. Japan's new dawn, *Popular Science and Technology,* [online] Available at:<http://www.popsci.com/popsci37b144110vgn/html> [Accessed 22 June 2009].

An intext reference for the above example would read:

(Kipper, 2008) ...

Journal Abstract from a Database

For a journal abstract from a database where you have been unable to access the full article, the required elements for a reference are:

Author, Initials., Year. Title of article. *Full Title of Journal,* [type of medium] Volume number (Issue/Part number), Page numbers if availalble, Abstract only.

Available through: [name of database]. [Accessed date].

Boughton, J.M., 2002. The Bretton Woods proposal: a brief look. Political Science Quarterly, [e-journal] 42(6), Abstract only. Available through: BlackwellScienceSynergy database [Accessed 12 June 2005].

Every effort should be made to read the article in full if you intend to use this work as supporting evidence in an academic submission.

Newspaper Articles

For newspaper articles the required elements for a reference are:

Author, Initials., Year. Title of article. *Full Title of Newspaper,* Day and month before page numbers and column line.

Slapper, G., 2005. Corporate manslaughter: new issues for lawyers. *The Times*, 3 Sep. p.4b.

(NB. 4b, this indicates that the article is on the fourth page of the newspaper, and "b" indicates this is the second column of newsprint across the page.)

Online Newspaper Articles

For newspaper articles found in online newspapers, the required elements for a reference are:

Author or corporate author, Year. Title of document or page. *Name of newspaper,* [type of medium] Additional date information. Available at:.[name of database]. [Accessed date].

Chittenden, M., Rogers, L. and Smith, D., 2003. Focus: 'Targetitis ails NHS. *Times Online,* [online]1 June. Available at: <http://www.timesonline.co.uk/tol/news/uk/scotland/article1138006.ece> [Accessed 17 March 2005].

Reference

Coney, J., 2009. Is this the start of a new home loan war? HSBC vows to lend £1billion to homebuyers with 10% deposits. *Daily Mail,* [online] (Last updated 9.47 AM on 09th April 2009) Available at: <http://www.dailymail.co.uk/news/article-1168461/Is-start-new-home-loan-war-HSBC-vows-lend-1billion-homebuyers-10-deposits.html> [Accessed on 20 April 2009].

An intext reference for the above example would read:

(Coney, 2009)

OTHER TYPES OF DOCUMENTS

There are other types of documents which you may wish to include in your reference list or bibliography. There is no official Harvard guide for these but some suggestions are set out below:

Acts of Parliament

The required elements are:

Short title with keywords capitalized, which includes the year followed by the chapter number in brackets. Keywords of titles are capitalized. Place of publication: Publisher.

Higher Education Act 2004. (c.8), London: HMSO.

For Acts prior to 1963, the regal year and parliamentary session are included:

Road Transport Lighting Act 1957. (5&6 Eliz. 2, c.51), London: HMSO.

If you need to refer to a specific section and paragraph, include the section, paragraph number and subsection.

Finance Act 2007. s.45(9)(b).

Statutory Instruments

The required elements for a reference are:

Short title (with key words capitalized). Year. the abbreviation 'SI' followed by the year of publication and the SI number. Place of publication: Publisher.

Public Offers of Securities Regulations 1995. SI 1995/1537, London: HMSO.

Official Publications such as Command Papers

The required elements for a reference are:

Authorship, which may be part of the title. Year. *Title, in italics if a separate element*, Offically assigned number such as a Command number as it is on the document, within brackets, Place of publication: Publisher.

Royal Commission on civil liability and compensation for personal injury, 1978. (Pearson Report) (Cmnd. 7054) London: HMSO.

Select Committee on nationalised industries (1978-9). *Consumers and the nationalised industries: prelegislative hearings* (HC 334 of 1978-9) London: HMSO.

Law Reports

It is recommended that you follow **accepted legal citation,** which is not part of the Harvard system. For this the required elements for a reference are:

Name of the parties involved in the law case, Year of reporting (in square brackets where there is no volume, or round brackets as indicated by the reference you are using) abbreviation for the law reporting series, part number/case number/page reference if available.

Jnes v Lipman [1962] 1 WLR 832.

Saidi v France (1994) 17 EHRR 251, p.245.

R v White (John Henry) [2005] EWCA Crim 689, 2005 WL 104528.

In the last example you should only quote the two law reports if you have used them.

An intext reference for the above example would read:

In the recent case of R v White (John Henry) (2005), the defence noted ...

Annual Report

The required elements for a reference are:

Corporate author, Year of publication. *Full title of annual report*, Place of Publication: Publisher.

Marks and Spencer, 2004. *The way forward, annual report 2003-2004*, London: Marks and Spencer.

For an **e-version** of an annual report. The required elements for a reference are:

Author or corporate author, Year. *Title of document or page*, [type of medium] Available at: include web site address/URL(Uniform Resource Locator) [Accessed date]

Marks and Spencer, 2004. *Annual report 2003-2004.* [Online] Available at: <http://www-marks-and-spencer.co.uk/corporate/annual2003/> [Accessed 4 June 2005].

Archive Material

If you have used material from Archives or Special collections, the required elements for a reference are:

Author, Initials., Year.*Title of document.* [type of medium]. Collection, Document number. Geographical Town/Place: Name of Library/Archive/Repository.

Brown, P.S., 1915. *An address to the Farmer.* [manuscript] Holdbury Collection. 600. London. Holdbury Library.

An intext reference for the above example would read:

(Brown, 1915)

British Standard and International Standards

The required elements for a reference are:

Corporate author, Year of Publication. *Identifying letters and numbers and full title of BS,* Place of publication: Publisher.

British Standards Institution, 1990. *BS 5555:1990 Recommendations for wiring identification.* Milton Keynes: BSI.

International Standards Office, 1998. ISO 690 - 2 *Information and documentation: Bibliographical references: Electronic documents.* Geneva: ISO.

Patent

The required elements for a reference are:

Inventor name, Initial(s)., Assignee.,Year.*Title.* Place. Patent number (status, if an application).

Example:

Graham, C.P., Fonti, L. and Martinez, A.M., 1972. *American Sugar Co. Tableting sugar and compositions containing it.* U.S. Pat. 3,642,535.

Leonard, Y., Super Sports Limited. 2008. *Tin can manufacture and method of sealing.* Canada. Pat. 12,789,675.

Conference Report

The required elements for a reference are:

Authorship/author, editor or organisation, Year. *Full title of conference report.* Location, Date, Place of publication: Publisher.

UNDESA (United Nations Department of Economic and Social Affairs), 2005. *6th Global forum on reinventing government: towards participatory and transparent governance.* Seoul, Republic of Korea 24-27 May 2005. New York: United Nations.

Conference Paper

The required elements for a reference are:

Authorship, Year. Full title of conference paper. In: followed by editor or name of organisation, *Full title of conference.* Location, Date, Place of publication: Publisher.

Brown, J., 2005. Evaluating surveys of transparent governance. In: UNDESA (United Nations Department of Economic and Social Affairs), *6th Global forum on reinventing government: towards participatory and transparent governance.* Seoul, Republic of Korea 24-27 May 2005. New York: United Nations.

Dissertation

The required elements for a reference are:

Author, Year of publication. *Title of dissertation*. Level. Official name of University.

Richmond, J., 2005. *Customer expectations in the world of electronic banking: a case study of the Bank of Britain*. Ph. D. Anglia Ruskin University.

DVD, Video or Film

The required elements for a reference are:

Full title of DVD or video. Year of release. [type of medium] Director. (if relevant) Country of origin: Film studio or maker. (Other relevant details).

Great films from the 80s: a selection of clips from Warner Brothers top films from the 1980s. 2005 [DVD] New York: Warner Brothers.

Health for all children 3: the video., 2004. [video] London: Child Growth Foundation. (Narrated by D.B.M. Hall).

For a film the suggested elements should include:

Title. Year of release. [Medium] Director. Country of origin: Film studio.

Macbeth, 1948. [Film] Directed by Orson Wells. USA: Republic Pictures.

Broadcasts

For a broadcast the suggested elements should include:

Series title and episode name and number if relevant, Year of broadcast. [type of medium] Broadcasting organisation and Channel, date and time of transmission.

Little Britain, 2006. [TV programme] BBC, BBC2, 30 January 2006 20.00.

EU Documents

Following EU conventions, examples of various EU documents are given below:

The required elements for a reference are:

The name of the Institution where the document originates (*e.g.* Commission) Form (*e.g.* Directive or Decision) Year/Legislation number/ Initials of Institution followed by the date it was passed if known, followed by the title, all in italics.

Council Directive 2001/29 /EC of 22 May 2001 on the harmonisation of certain aspects of copyright and related rights in the information society.

Commission Decision 93/42/EEC of 21 December 1992 concerning additional guarantees relating to infectious bovine rhinotracheitis for bovines destined for Denmark.

EU Regulation 1408/71
REGULATION (EEC) No 1408/71 OF THE COUNCIL of 14 June 1971 on the application of social security schemes to employed persons and their families moving within the Community.

Council Regulation (EEC) 1612/68[5] of 15 October 1968 on freedom of movement for workers within the Community.

Course Material

It is important to check with the lecturer who has given the lecture that they are in agreement with course material being included in any Reference List. If they are in agreement, and if it is not a publicly available document, it is important to provide a copy in the Appendix of your work. The citation to the course material in your Reference List should then also refer to the Appendix.

It would also be advisable to follow up any sources mentioned in your lecture and read these for yourself.

Course Material/Lecture Notes – Print Version

The required elements for a reference are:

Lecturer/Author, initial. Year. 'Title of item', *Module Code Module title.* HE Institution, unpublished.

Williams, B., 2008. Guide to project management, *BD45001S Management.* Anglia Ruskin University, unpublished.

An intext reference for the above example would read:

(Williams, 2008)

Course Material – Electronic

The required elements for a reference are:

Lecturer/Author name, initial. Year. 'Title of item', *Module Code Module Title* [online via internal VLE], HE Institution. Available at:

web address if available over the internet, otherwise indicate if available through WebCT, SharePoint or other virtual learning environment address.
[Accessed date].

Williams, B., 2008. Guide to project management, BD45001S Management. [online via internal VLE] Anglia Ruskin University Available at:< J:\AIBS\AIBS Admin\ASSESSMENT MATERIAL\ASSESSMENT MATERIAL 2009-10\IBS and MARKETING and MA ARTS\IBS Sem 2 2009-10 Approved Material\Sem 2> [Accessed Date 13 June 2008].

An intext reference for the above examples would read:

(Williams, 2008) ...

Map

The required elements for a reference are:

Map maker, Year of issue. Title of map. *Map series*, Sheet number, scale, Place of publication: Publisher.

Ordnance Survey, 2006. Chester and North Wales. *Landranger series*, Sheet 106, 1:50000, Southampton: Ordnance Survey.

Quotations from Written Plays

When reviewing a number of different plays it is essential to cite the title of the plays. If reviewing one play (for example Twelfth Night) it is not necessary to repeat the title in your citations.

Published plays may contain line numbers, particularly in classic texts such as Shakespeare. If they exist it is good practice to include the line number, but Act and Scene numbers must always be included.

Classic plays are available in edited editions and the editor's name should be included with your reference.

The required elements for a reference are:

Author, Initials., Year (of the edition). *Title of play.* Editors, Edition. (only include this if not the first edition) Place of publication: (this must be a town or city, not a country) Publisher.

Shakespeare, W. 1995. *Twelfth Night,* (World's Classics series) Warren, R and Wells, T. eds. Oxford: Oxford University Press

An intext reference for the above examples would read:

Much speculation has occurred when Malvolio imagines he might marry Olivia, *"there is example for't; the Lady of the Strachy married the yeoman of the wardrobe"* (Shakespeare, Twelfth Night Act 2 Scene 5 Line no 36-7).

Pictures, Images and Photographs

The suggested elements for a reference are:

Artist/Photographer's name (if known), Year of production. *Title of image.* [type of medium] Collection Details as available (Collection, Document number, Geographical Town/Place: Name of Library/Archive/Repository).

Beaton,C., 1956. *Marilyn Monroe.* [photograph] (Marilyn Monroe's own private collection).

Beaton,C., 1944. China 1944: *A mother resting her head on her sick child's pillow in the Canadian Mission Hospital in Chengtu.* [photograph] (Imperial War Museum Collection).

For an electronic reference the suggested elements are:

Artist/Photographer's name, Year of production. *Title of image.* [type of medium] Available at: include web site address/ URL(Uniform Resource Locator) and additional details of access, such as the routing from the homepage of the source.[Accessed date].

Dean, R, 2008 *Tales from Topographic Oceans.* [electronic print] Available at: <http://rogerdean.com/store/product_info.php?cPath=4&products_id=88> [Accessed 18 June 2008].

Interviews

Where you have conducted an interview - from a primary source

Where you are conducting the interview, it is important to check with the person being interviewed that they will be in agreement with a transcript of the interview being made available. Since this will not be a publicly available document, it may be included as a transcript within an Appendix in your piece of work.

The citation for this interview should refer to the Appendix.

In an interview (Appendix A) the findings of the report were reviewed and White agreed with ...

In the Appendix you should include details such as:

Interviewee's name. Year of interview. *Title of interview..* Interviewed by ...name. [type of medium/format] Location and exact date of interview . Together with the transcript.

The suggested elements for a reference are:

Interviewee name, and initial(s)., Year of Interview. *Title of Interview (or Interview on ..name of programme)* Interviewed by ...name. [type of medium/format] Name of Channel, Date of transmission, time of transmission.

Ahern, B., 1999. *Interview on Morning Ireland* Interviewed by... John Boyd [radio] RTE Radio 1, 15 February 1999, 08:30.

An intext reference for the above examples would read:

(Ahern, 1999)

Press release

These may be paper or electronic.

For a paper resource

Corporate author of press release, Year. *Title.* Press release and date.

RCN, 2009. RCN praises health care staff as infections continue to fall. Press release, 18 June 2009.

Electronic

Corporate author of press release, Year. *Title.* [press release] date, Available at: web address [Accessed date].

RCN, 2009. RCN praises health care staff as infections continue to fall. [press release] 18 June 2009, Available at:<http://www.rcn.org.uk/newsevents/news/article/uk/rcn_praises_health_care_staff_as_infections_continue_to_fall> [Accessed 23 June 2009].

ELECTRONIC SOURCES

Websites

For websites found on the worldwide web the required elements for a reference are:

Authorship or Source, Year. *Title of web document* or web page. [type of medium] (date of update if available) Available at: include web site address/URL (Uniform Resource Locator) [Accessed date].

If the URL appears to be exceedingly long, provide routing details which enable the reader to access the particular page via the site's homepage. You may be taken to a particular page as a result of a search you performed, or be directed from a link to another place on a website. The resultant URLs may include specific data about your method of accessing that page that is not available to your reader. If this is the case use the homepage (from which the reference can be found).

Static URL

NHS Evidence, 2003. *National Library of Guidelines.* [online] Available at: <http://www.library.nhs.uk/guidelinesFinder> [Accessed 10 October 2009].

Dynamic URL

We have highlighted the part of the URL that shows this is a dynamic search. If this is not available to everyone, use the second example below:

Example 1

National Electronic Library for Health, 2003. *Can walking make you slimmer and healthier?* (Hitting the headlines article) [online] (Updated 16 Jan 2005) Available at: <http://www.library.nhs.uk/rss/newsAndRssArticle.aspx?uri=http%3A%2F%2Fwww. .library.nhs.uk %2Fresources%2F%3Fid%3D66149> [Accessed 10 April 2005].

Example 2

National Electronic Library for Health, 2003. *Can walking make you slimmer and healthier?* (Hitting the headlines article) [online] (Updated 16 Jan 2005) Available at: <http://www.library.nhs.uk> [Accessed 10 April 2005].

The title of a web page is normally the main heading on the page, or the title displayed on the top of the web browser.

An intext reference for the above examples would read.

(National Electronic Library for Health, 2003)

Publications Available from Websites

For publications found on the internet the required elements for a reference are:

Author or corporate author, Year. *Title of document.* [type of medium] Place: Producer/Publisher. Available at: include website address/URL(Uniform Resource Locator).[Accessed date].

Scottish Intercollegiate Guidelines, 2001. *Hypertension in the elderly.* (SIGN publication 20) [online] Edinburgh : SIGN (Published 2001) Available at: <http://www.sign.ac.uk/pdf/sign49.pdf [Accessed 17 March 2005].

Boots Group Plc., 2003. *Corporate social responsibility.* [online] Boots Group Plc. Available at: <http://www.Boots-Plc.Com/Information/Info.Asp?Level1id=447&Level 2id=0> [Accessed 23 July 2005].

Defoe, D., 1999. *The fortunes and the misfortunes of the famous Moll Flanders.* [online] Champaign, Illinois: Project Gutenberg. Available at: <http://www.gutenberg.org/etext/370> [Accessed 18 November 2005].

Independent Inquiry into Access to Healthcare for People with Learning Disabilities. n.d. Healthcare for all. [online] Available at: <http://www.iahpld.org.uk/Healthcare_easy_final.pdf> [Accessed 10 April 2009]

Electronic Images

For images found on the internet the required elements for a reference are:

Author, Year (image created). *Title of work.* [type of medium] Available at: include website address/URL (Uniform Resource Locator) [Accessed date].

Where the author is not known, begin the reference with the *title of the work.*

Where none of the usual details are known, (such as author, date, or image title) try to find the filename of the image (for example by right clicking and looking at the properties of the file). If none of the above is available begin the reference with the *subject and title of the work.*

Van Vechten, C. 1934. *Man Ray.* [photograph] Available at: <http://en.wikipedia.org/wiki/File:Man_Ray_1934.jpg> [Accessed 04 October 2009].

Pepsi, 2009. *Pepsi can designs.* [image online] Available at: <http://www.pepsi.co.uk/MaxYourPepsi.aspx> [Accessed 19 June 2009].

[Nimbus 1 returned sharp cloud cover photos, plus night time infra red pictures] n.d. [image online] Available at: <http://rammb.cira.colostate.edu/dev/hillger/Nimbus-1_image.jpg> [Accessed 13 November 2008].

[Child placing gauze over knee wound] n.d. [image online] Available at: < http://www.dadpal.com/2009/12/wounds-care-help-and-wound-vac-therapy.html> [Accessed 01 June 2010].

An in text reference for the above examples would read:

(Van Vechten, 1934)

(Pepsi, 2009)

(Nimbus 1, n.d.)

(Child placing gauze, n.d.)

E-mail Correspondence/Discussion Lists

For e-mail correspondence or discussion lists the suggested elements for a reference are:

Name of sender and e-mail address, Year. *Message or subject title from posting line.* [type of medium] Recipient's name and e-mail address. Date sent: Including time. Available at: URL (e.g. details of where message is archived). [Accessed date].

Jones, P., jones@jones.com, 2005. *Mobile phone developments.* [email] Message to R G. Schmit (r.g.schmit@syy.ac.uk). Sent Monday 7 June 2005, 08:13. Available at: <http://gog.defer.com/2004_07_01_defer_archive.html> [Accessed 7 July 2005].

Blogs

The required elements for a reference are:

Author, Year. Title of individual blog entry. *Blog title,* [medium] Blog posting date. Available at: include website address/URL (Uniform Resource Locator) [Accessed date].

Whitton Felix, 2009. Conservationists are not making themselves heard. *Guardian.co.uk Science blog,* [blog] 18 June, Available at:

<http://www.guardian.co.uk/science/blog/2009/jun/18/conservation-extinction-open-ground> [Accessed 23 June 2009].

Blog Comments

The required elements for a reference are:

Comment Author, Year. Title of individual blog entry. *Blog title,* [medium] Comment posting date. Available at: include website address/URL (Uniform Resource Locator) [Accessed date].

DGeezer, 2009. Conservationists are not making themselves heard. *Guardian.co.uk Science blog,* [blog] 18 June, Available at: <http://www.guardian.co.uk/science/blog/2009/jun/18/conservation-extinction-open-ground> [Accessed 23 June 2009].

An in text reference for the above examples would read:

(Whitton, 2009)

(Geezer, 2009)

Mailing List

The required elements for a reference are:

Author, Initial., Year. Subject Line, *Title of Mailing List.* [online] date of message, Available at: include website address/URL (Uniform Resource Locator) [Accessed date].

Murrey, T., 2009. 'Sharing good practice', *Forum for International Students.* [online] 23 June 2009, Available at : <http://www.internationalstudentforum.com> [Accessed 23 June 2009].

Podcast or Archived TV Programme

The required elements for a reference are:

Broadcaster/Author, Year. *Programme title,* Series Title. (if relevant) [type of medium] date of transmission. Available at: include web site address/URL (Uniform Resource Locator) [Accessed date].

National Gallery, 2008. *Episode Seventeen (March 2008),* The National Gallery Monthly Podcast. [podcast] March 2008. Available at: < http://www.nationalgallery.org.uk/podcasts> [Accessed 23 June 2009].

You Tube video

The required elements for a reference are:

Screen name of contributor,Year. *Video Title,* Series Title. (if relevant) [type of medium] Available at: include web site address/ URL (Uniform Resource Locator) [Accessed date].

Mrgeorged, 2009. *Top Gear The Stig revealed Full.* [video online] Available at:<http://www.youtube.com/watch#!v= eTapK5dRaw4> [Accessed 23 June 2009].

UNPUBLISHED WORKS

Unpublished Works

You may occasionally have access to a document before it is published and may therefore not be able to provide full details:

Bloggs, J., (in press) *A new book that I have written.* London: Vanity Press

Woolley, E. and Muncey, T., (in press) Demons or diamonds: a study to ascertain the range of attitudes present in health professionals to children with conduct disorder. *Journal of Adolescent Psychiatric Nursing.* (Accepted for publication December 2002).

Informal or In-house Publications

For informal publications, such as class handouts and leaflets, provide what details you can:

Anglia Ruskin University, 2007. *Using the Cochrane Library.* [leaflet] August 2007 ed. Cambridge: Anglia Ruskin University.

Personal Communication

Where you refer to a more informal personal communication, *e.g.* letter, e-mail, phone call or conversation, provide as much detail as possible and note the nature of the communication:

Permission should be sought before these sources are quoted, and a copy retained for reference.

Hindle, E., 2000. *Introducing Cow and Gate Omneo Comfort: an infant milk for digestive comfort.* [letter] (Personal communication, 2 June 2000).

O'Sullivan, S., 2003. *Discussion on citation and referencing.* [letter] (Personal communication, 5 June 2003).

5.4.2 AMERICAN PSYCHOLOGICAL ASSOCIATION (APA) (http://en.wikipedia.org/wiki/APA_style)

Summary

APA (American Psychological Association) is most commonly used to cite sources within the social sciences. This resource, revised according to the 6th edition, second printing of the APA manual, offers examples for the general format of APA research papers, in-text citations, endnotes/footnotes, and the reference page.

APA Style has been adapted by many disciplines and is used by writers around the world. The *Publication Manual of the American Psychological Association* is the style manual of choice for writers, editors, students, and educators in the social and behavioral sciences. It provides invaluable guidance on all aspects of the writing process, from the ethics of authorship to the word choice that best reduces bias in language

CITATIONS

APA uses two methods to cite the use of a source in an essay's text: parenthetical citation and attribution in the text of the essay. Page numbers are not required in APA in-text citation but are recommended.

In-Text Citations

The general format for attribution within your text is:Author Last Name (Year of Publication) has argued this point.

Example: Smith (1988) has argued this point.

Example: Smith (1988, p. 244) has written that... or Smith (1988) has written that...

Parenthetical Citations

The general format for parenthetical citations in APA style is: (Author Last Name, Year of Publication) Example: (Smith, 1988)

APA Citation Examples

Based on APA Publication Manual 6th edition, 2009

Reference List Examples

Articles

- Academic Journals
- Magazines

- ☆ Newspapers
- ☆ Encyclopaedia Articles
- ☆ Articles Freely Available on the Web
- ☆ Book, Film, and Product Reviews
- ☆ Books
- ☆ E-books
- ☆ Websites
- ☆ WebTycho Classroom Materials
- ☆ Technical and Research Reports
- ☆ Dissertations and Theses
- ☆ Images
- ☆ Interviews, E-mail Messages, and Other Personal Communications

General Rules

In-Text citations

What you are Citing	*In-Text Citations*
The entire work	(Smith, 2004)
A specific page	(Smith, 2004, p. 39)
If the author's name is included in the text of the sentence where the citation takes place	Smith (2004, p. 39) claims that... Use only the date or date and page number.
An online article with no page numbers	(Myers, 2000, para. 5) (Beutler, 2000, Conclusion section, para. 1) Use abbreviation "para." followed by the paragraph number you are citing. When possible, specify a section of the article.
Citing multiple authors	See Authors, below.

Authors

One Author

Example: Reference List Citation	*Example: In-Text Citation*
Courtois, C. A. (2004).	(Courtois, 2004)

Two Authors

Example: Reference List Citation	*Example: In-Text Citation*
Kelley, P. C., and Chang, P. L. (2007)	(Kelley and Chang, 2007)

Three to Five Authors

Example: Reference List Citation	*Example: In-Text Citation*
Hughes, J. C., Brestan, E. V., and Valle, L. A. (2004).	**First citation:** (Hughes, Brestan, and Valle, 2004) **Subsequent citations:** (Hughes *et al.*, 2004) When a work has more than 2 authors, subsequent in-text citations consist of the first author's name followed by "*et al.*" (Latin for "and others") and the date.

Six or Seven Authors

Example: Reference List Citation	*Example: In-Text Citation*
Phelps, B. R., Lima, M., Gomez, J., MacArthur, R. T., Gansu, L., & Nehru, M. (2004).	**First citation:** (Phelps *et al.*, 2004)

Example: Reference List Citation	*Example: In-Text Citation*
	Subsequent citations: (Phelps *et al.*, 2004)
	When a work has 6-7 authors, in-text citations consist of the first author's name followed by "*et al.*" (Latin for "and others") and the date.

Eight or more Authors

Example: Reference List Citation	*Example: In-Text Citation*
Carter, A., Dougherty, S., Addington, M., Stanley, R., Stanley, C., Schuffler, G., . . . Smyrna, B. F. (2004).	**First citation:** (Carter *et al.*, 2004)
When there are eight or more authors, include the first 6 authors' names followed by an ellipsis (. . .) and the final author's name.	**Subsequent citations:** (Carter *et al.*, 2004) When a work has 8 or more authors, in-text citations consist of the first author's name followed by "*et al.*" (Latin for "and others") and the date.

Group Author

Example: Reference List Citation	*Example: In-Text Citation*
American Dietetic Association (1999)	**First citation:** (American Dietetic Association [ADA], 1999) **Subsequent citations:** (ADA, 1999)

No Authors Listed

Example: Reference List Citation	*Example: In-Text Citation*
None to claim their bones: Relics of an old Brooklyn graveyard. (1888, April 12). *New York Times*, pp. 3-4. Retrieved from http://www.nytimes.com/	("None to Claim Their Bones," 1888)
	In cases where the title contains a colon, use only the text before the colon in your in-text citation.
List the source by title in your reference list. Alphabetize reference list entries beginning with a title using the primary word of the title (excluding *a*, *an*, and *the*).	

Titles

Capitalization

For all sources other than periodicals (that is, newspapers, magazines, and scholarly journals), capitalize the first word of the title and subtitle and proper nouns only. Do not capitalize the rest (see example below).

All major words in periodical titles should be capitalized (for example, *Psychology Today*, *Journal of Health Care for the Poor and Underserved*.)

Italics: Titles are italicized for the following items:

- ☆ Books
- ☆ E-Books
- ☆ Periodicals
- ☆ Websites
- ☆ Dissertations/theses
- ☆ Reports/technical papers
- ☆ Works of art

Source	*Example*
Journal article title	Freud's *Vienna* revisited.
Book title	*Student cheating and plagiarism in the Internet era: A wake-up call.*

Volume and Issue Numbers

APA does not use "Volume", "Vol.", "v.", "Issue" or related terms. Use italics for the volume number.

Source	*Example*
Magazine and journal volume	*12*(4)
and issue number formatting	12 is the volume number (in italics) and 4 is the issue number.
	If each issue of a journal begins on page 1, give the issue number in parentheses immediately after the volume number, as above.

Page Numbers

Undated Sources

Use "(n.d.)" (for "no date") in your citation.

Reference List of Citation	*In-Text Citation*
Knowles, A. (n.d.). *House of dust* [Collage]. Whitney Museum of American Art, New York. Retrieved from Oxford Art Online database.	(Knowles, n.d.)

Citing a Source within a Source

Scenario: You read a 2007 article by Linhares and Brum that cites an earlier article, by Frederick. You want to cite Frederick's article, but you have not read Frederick's article itself.

Reference List of Citation	*In-Text Citation*
Linhares, A., and Brum, P. (2007). Understanding our understanding of strategic scenarios: What role do chunks play? *Cognitive Science, 31*(6), 989-1007. doi:10.1080/03640210701703725 Your Reference list will contain the article you read, by Linhares and Brum. Your Reference list will NOT contain a citation for Frederick's article.	Frederick's study (as cited in Linhares and Brum, 2007) found that... Your in-text citation gives credit to Frederick and shows the source in which you found Frederick's ideas.

Articles

Academic Journals

Source	*Reference List Citation*
Library database with DOI	Sagarin, B. J., and Lawler-Sagarin, K. A. (2005). Critically evaluating competing theories: An exercise based on the Kitty Genovese murder. *Teaching of Psychology, 32*(3), 167–169. doi:10.1207/s15328023top3203_8 **What is a DOI?** Some library databases, such as PsycARTICLES and PsycINFO, list a Digital Object Identifier (DOI) for individual articles. A DOI is a unique identifying number for an article. In the database record for an article, you will see an element that looks like this, which you should include at the end of your APA reference:

Source	*Reference List Citation*
Library database without DOI	Reitzes, D. C., and Mutran, E. J. (2004). The transition to retirement: Stages and factors that influence retirement adjustment. *International Journal of Aging and Human Development, 59*(1), 63-84. Retrieved from http://www.baywood.com/journals/PreviewJournals.asp?Id=0091-4150
	No DOI? Find the journal homepage. Do a Web search (using a search engine such as Google or Yahoo!) to find the address of the homepage of the journal that published the article and include it in your citation (example). Please be aware, however, that the full text of articles may not actually be available at the journal homepage.
	Cannot find the journal homepage? In this case, do a Web search (using a search engine such as Google or Yahoo!) for the name of the database you are using (for example, "JSTOR" or "Business Source Complete") and use the address of its homepage.
Free Web	Giancola, P. R. (2004). Executive functioning and alcohol-related aggression. *American Psychologist, 59*(2), 5-7. Retrieved from http://www.apa.org/journals/amp/
In print	Hughes, J. C., Brestan, E. V., and Valle, L. A. (2004). Problem-solving interactions between mothers and children. *Child and Family Behavior Therapy, 26*(1), 1-16.

Magazines

Daily or Weekly Magazines

Source	*Reference List Citation*
Library database	Borowitz, A. (2004, November 15). Pavlov's brother. *New Yorker, 80*(35), 63-66. Retrieved from http://www.newyorker.com/
	Do a Web search (using a search engine such as Google or Yahoo!) for the magazine homepage and use the homepage URL after the words "Retrieved from".
Free Web	Springen, K. (2005, January 17). Artful aging. *Newsweek, 145*(3), 25-27. Retrieved from http://www.newsweek.com/
In print	Borowitz, A. (2004, November 15). Pavlov's brother. *New Yorker, 80*(35), 63-66.

Monthly Magazines

Source	*Reference List Citation*
Library database	Norman, A. D. (1988, March). Infuriating by design.*Psychology Today, 22*(3), 52-56. Retrieved from http://www.psychologytoday.com/
	Do a Web search (using a search engine such as Google or Yahoo!) for the magazine homepage and use the homepage URL after the words "Retrieved from".
Free Web	Gelb, N. (2003, May). Winter of discontent. *Smithsonian, 34*(2), 50-55. Retrieved from http://www.smithsonianmagazine.com/
In print	Ives, F., and Lydon, J. (2005, January). Freud's Vienna revisited. *Discover, 26*(2), 16-17.

Tip

☆ When an issue of a magazine covers several months, the name of the first and last month in the range should be given in the citation, separated by a dash, for example: "(1993, June-July)".

Newspapers

Source	*Reference List Citation*
Library database	Brown, P. L. (1999, September 5). Tiffany glass and other tales from the crypt. *The New York Times*, pp. 1, 5. Retrieved from http://www.nytimes.com/
	Do a Web search (using a search engine such as Google or Yahoo!) for the newspaper homepage and use the homepage URL after the words "Retrieved from".
Free Web	Foreman, J. (2003, August 12). Allston gothic. *The Boston Globe*. Retrieved from http://www.boston.com/
In print	Brown, P. L. (1999, September 5). Tiffany glass and other tales from the crypt. *The New York Times*, pp. 1, 5.
	The page number of a newspaper article is preceded by"**p.**" in a reference list citation. When an article appears on multiple pages, the page range is preceded by "**pp.**"(for example, "pp. 4-6"). When an article appears on discontinuous pages, separate the page numbers with a comma (ex. "pp. 4, 8"). When a newspaper uses section letters in its page numbers, these should be included in your citation (ex. "p. A1", "pp. B1, B6").

Encyclopaedia Articles

Source	*Reference List Citation*
Library database	Smith, A. J. (2001). Child development. In B. Strickland (Ed.), *The Gale encyclopaedia of psychology*. Retrieved from http://www.gale.cengage.com/ Do a Web search (using a search engine such as Google or Yahoo!) for the homepage of the publisher of the encyclopaedia and use the homepage URL after the words "Retrieved from".

Articles Freely Available on the Web

Source	*Reference List Citation*
Free Web	Caliper, N. (2004). The Brontes and the world they made.*The Victorian Web*. Retrieved from http://www.victorians.org/bronte.html

Book, Film and Product Reviews

Source	*Reference List Citation*
Library database	Grimes, W. (2006, December 13). Beyond Mandalay, the road to isolation and xenophobia [Review of the book *The river of lost footsteps: Histories of Burma*, by T. Myint-U]. *New York Times*, pp. E8, E10. Retrieved from http://www.nytimes.com/ Do a Web search (using a search engine such as Google or Yahoo!) for the newspaper homepage and use the homepage URL after the words "Retrieved from". **An untitled book, film, or product review (for example, a review covering multiple works):**

Source	*Reference List Citation*
	Guha, M. (2006). [Review of the books *Fleeting pleasures: A history of intoxicants,* by M. London and *Dirty: A search for answers inside America's teenage drug epidemic*, by M. Maran]. *Journal of Mental Health, 15,* 713-716. Retrieved from http://www.informaworld.com/smpp/title~content=t713432595
	Do a Web search (using a search engine such as Google or Yahoo!) for the journal homepage and use the homepage URL after the words "Retrieved from".
Free Web	Cohen, P. (2007, May 9). Love, honor, cherish, and buy [Review of the book *One perfect day: The selling of the American wedding*,by R. Mead]. *New York Times*. Retrieved from http://www.nytimes.com/2007/05/09/books/09bride.html

Books

Source	*Reference List Citation*
Basic book	Jans, N. (1993). *The last light breaking: Life among Alaska's Inupiat Eskimos*. Anchorage, AK: Alaska Northwest Books.
Edited book	Miller, J., and Smith, T. (Eds.). (1996). *Cape Cod stories: Tales from Cape Cod, Nantucket, and Martha's Vineyard*. San Francisco, CA: Chronicle Books.
	For a single editor, use "(Ed.)".
Numbered edition other than the first	Arking, R. (2006). *The biology of aging: Observations and principles* (3rd ed.). New York, NY: Oxford University Press.
Revised edition	Culliney, J. L. (2006). *Islands in a far sea: The fate of nature in Hawai'i* (Rev. ed.). Honolulu, HI: University of Hawai'i Press.

Source	*Reference List Citation*
Multi-volume set	Green, C. M. (1962-1963). *Washington* (Vols. 1-2). Princeton, NJ: Princeton University Press.
	If volumes in a work or set are published in different years, give the range of years separated by a dash as above.
Chapter or article in an anthology	Eliot, T. S. (2001). Tradition and the individual talent. In V. B. Leitch (Ed.), *The Norton anthology of theory and criticism* (pp. 1092-1097). New York, NY: W. W. Norton. (Original work published 1920)
	Note that the page numbers of an article or chapter are preceded by "pp." when citing it (for example, "pp. 25-50"). In cases where an article/chapter occupies a single page, the page is preceded by "p." (ex. "p. 4").
	If an article has been reprinted from a source published earlier, give the original date of publication in the "original work" element of the citation as shown above (when using this element, *the final period in a citation is omitted*).

Tips

- ☆ **Cities, States and Countries:** For U.S. cities, add the standard postal abbreviations for state (for example, "Chatham, MA"). Foreign cities should be followed by the name of their country (ex. "Brisbane, Australia").
- ☆ **Place of publication:** Separate place of publication from publisher with a colon (for example "New York, NY: Zone Books"). If more than one city is given, list only the first.
- ☆ **Publisher names:** "Co.", "Inc." and related abbreviations should not be included in citations (for example, "Ivan R. Dee, Inc." should be given as "Ivan R. Dee".)

E-Books

Source	*Reference List Citation*
Net Library	Kornblum, W. (2002). *At sea in the city: New York from the water's edge*. Chapel Hill, NC: Algonquin Books. Retrieved from http://www.workman.com/algonquin/
	Do a Web search (using a search engine such as Google or Yahoo!) for the homepage of the publisher of the book and use the homepage URL after the words "Retrieved from".
Free Web	Seton, E. T. (1911). *The Arctic prairies: A canoe-journey of 2,000 miles in search of the caribou*. New York, NY: C. Scribner's Sons. Retrieved from Project Gutenberg: http://www.gutenberg.org/etext/6818
Book chapter from a library database (suggested format)	Quina, K., and Kanarian, M A. (1988). Continuing education. In R. Shepard and M. Herlong (Eds.), *Teaching a psychology of people: Resources for gender and sociocultural awareness* (pp. 200-208). Washington, DC: American Psychological Association. Retrieved from http://www.apa.org/
	Do a Web search (using a search engine such as Google or Yahoo!) for the homepage of the publisher of the book and use the homepage URL after the words "Retrieved from".
	Library databases may include chapters from books. Information about the publisher of a book can often be found in the description of the chapter in the database. Author and publisher information may be omitted from your citation if it is not available.

Tips

- ☆ **Cities, States and Countries:** For U.S. cities, add the standard postal abbreviations for state (for example, "Chatham, MA"). Foreign cities should be followed by the name of their country (ex. "Brisbane, Australia").
- ☆ **Place of publication:** Separate place of publication from publisher with a colon (for example "New York, NY: Zone Books"). If more than one city is given, list only the first.
- ☆ **Publisher names:** "Co.", "Inc." and related abbreviations should not be included in citations (for example, "Ivan R. Dee, Inc." should be given as "Ivan R. Dee".

Websites

Source	*Reference List Citation*
Entire Website	If you refer to an entire Website, you do not need to include an entry for it in your reference list, but must identify the source clearly in the text of your paper. For example: The Sea Turtle Restoration Project homepage presents a wealth of compelling, well-researched information on the struggle to save the world's sea turtles from extinction (http://www.seaturtles.org).
A specific page within a Website	Sea Turtle Restoration Project. (2006). *Threats to sea turtles*. Retrieved from http://seaturtles.org/section.php?id=104 **In-text Citation:** (Sea Turtle Restoration Project, 2006)

WebTycho Classroom Materials

Source	*Reference List Citation*
A document in a WebTycho classroom	Whitford, D. (2006). *Cross-curricular initiatives in NSCI170*. Document posted in University of Maryland University College

Source	*Reference List Citation*
	NSCI 170 6981 online classroom, archived at: http://webtycho.umuc.edu
	No official APA format for citing online classroom materials exists - this is merely a recommended format to use in citing such documents.

Technical and Research Report

Source	*Reference List Citation*
Free Web	United States General Accounting Office. (1997, February). *Telemedicine: Federal strategy is needed to guide investments* (Publication No. GAO/NSAID/HEHS-97-67). Retrieved from General Accounting Office Reports Online: www.gpoaccess.gov/gaoreports/ index.html
In print	United States General Accounting Office. (1997, February). *Telemedicine: Federal strategy is needed to guide investments* (Publication No. GAO/NSAID/HEHS-97-67). Washington, DC: U.S. Government Printing Office.

Tip

- ☆ The element of the citation giving the publication or report number can be omitted if this information is not available for the source you're citing.

Dissertations and Theses

Dissertations

Source	*Reference List Citation*
Dissertations and Theses database	Pecore, J. T. (2004). *Sounding the spirit of Cambodia: The living tradition of Khmer music and dance-drama in a Washington, DC*

Source	Reference List Citation
	community (Doctoral dissertation). Retrieved from Dissertations and Theses database. (UMI No. 3114720) Note that a "Retrieved from" statement is used, giving the database name followed by the word "database." Also, APA calls for the citation to end with a unique identifying number for the dissertation, labeling it "UMI No." That number can be found in Dissertations and Theses database, listed in the item record as "Publication Number."
Free Web	Caprette, C. L. (2005). *Conquering the cold shudder: The origin and evolution of snake eyes* (Doctoral dissertation). Retrieved from http://www.ohiolink.edu/etd/send-pdf.cgi?acc_num=osu1111184984
In print	Caprette, C. L. (2005). *Conquering the cold shudder: The origin and evolution of snake eyes* (Doctoral dissertation). Ohio State University, Columbus, OH.

Master's Theses

Source	Reference List Citation
Dissertations and Theses database	Harzbecker, J. J. (1999). *Life and death in Washington DC: An analysis of the Mortality Census data of 1850* (Master's thesis). Retrieved from Dissertations and Theses database. (UMI No. 1395513) Note that a "Retrieved from" statement is used, giving the database name followed by the word "database." Also, APA calls for the citation to end with a unique identifying number for the dissertation,

Source	*Reference List Citation*
	labeling it "UMI No." That number can be found in Dissertations and Theses database, listed in the item record as "Publication Number."
Free Web	Angelova, A. N. (2004). *Data pruning* (Master's thesis). Retrieved from http://resolver.caltech.edu/CaltechETD:etd-05282004-000943
In print	Angelova, A. N. (2004). *Data pruning* (Master's thesis). California Institute of Technology, Pasadena, CA.

Images

Titled Image

Source	*Reference List Citation*
Library database	Rousseau, H. (1896). *The ship in the storm* [Painting]. Musee de l'Orangerie, Paris. Retrieved from Oxford Art Online database.
Free Web	Rousseau, H. (1896). *The ship in the storm* [Painting]. Musee de l'Orangerie, Paris. Retrieved from http://www.uwm.edu/~wash/rousseau.jpg
Image reproduced in a printed source	Rousseau, H. (1896). *The ship in the storm* [Painting]. Musee de l'Orangerie, Paris. *Henri Rousseau: Jungles in Paris*. By Claire Fresches *et al*. Washington, DC: National Gallery of Art. 232. The plate/image number (or, if this number is not available, the page number on which the image is printed) should follow the name of the publisher as shown.

Untitled Image

Create a brief title for it and place it in brackets, unitalicized.

Source	*Reference List Citation*
Library database	Muybridge, E. [Photograph of a horse running]. (1887). National Gallery, London. Retrieved from Academic Search Complete database.
Image reproduced in a printed source	Muybridge, E. [Photograph of a horse running]. (1887). National Gallery, London. *River of shadows: Eadweard Muybridge and the technological wild West*. By Rebecca Solnit. New York, NY: Viking. 52.
	The plate/image number (or, if this number is not available, the page number on which the image is printed) should follow the name of the publisher as shown.

Tips

☆ **Medium:** If known, the medium of the image should be placed in brackets as shown above, and the collection which owns the image included in your citation along with its location.

☆ **Institution locations:** For U.S. cities, add the standard postal abbreviations for state (for example, "Chatham, MA"). Foreign cities should be followed by the name of their country (ex. "Brisbane, Australia").

Interviews, E-mail messages, and other Personal Communications

Source	*Examples*
Personal communication	APA does not require that you cite personal communications (interviews you've conducted, e-mail messages, etc.) in your reference list. instead, give an in-text citation only using the following model:
	Joe Smith (personal communication, November 18, 2006) informed me that the server had crashed several hours ago.

BOOK

Geissler, E. M. (1998). *Pocket guide to cultural assessment* (2nd ed.). St. Louis, MO: Mosby.

You can also go to WorldCat.org, search the world's largest database of library books, and click on "Cite this item" for almost any book. Its APA citations are not 100% correct, though; beware of capitalization, state of publication, and punctuation errors (see NOTES).

BOOK CHAPTER, ESSAY, or ARTICLE when Author is Credited

de Paula, T. C. M., Lagana, K., and Gonzalez-Ramirez, L. (1996). Mexican Americans. In J. G. Lipson, S. L Dibble, and P. A. Minarik (Eds.), *Culture and nursing care: A pocket guide* (pp. 203-221). San Francisco: USCF Nursing Press.

ARTICLE OR CHAPTER IN EDITED BOOK

Ruiz, V. L. (1992). Star struck: Acculturation, adolescence, and Mexican American women, 1920-1950. In E. West and P. Petrik (Eds.), *Small worlds: Children and adolescents in Lawrence, America, 1850-1950* (pp.118-224). Plains, KS: University Press of Kansas.

BOOK CHAPTER, ESSAY, or ARTICLE when No Author is Credited (Paper version)

Russians. (1998). In T. L. Gall (Ed.), *Worldmark encyclopaedia of cultures and daily life* (Vol. 4, pp. 332-339). Detroit, MI: Gale Research.

BOOK CHAPTER, ESSAY, or ARTICLE when No Author is Credited (Online version)

Russians. (1998). *Worldmark encyclopaedia of cultures and daily life*. Retrieved January 9, 2003 from Discovering Collection database.

ARTICLE in a STANDARD ENCYCLOPAEDIA (Paper copy)

Islam. (1992). In *The new encyclopaedia Britannica* (Vol. 22, pp. 1-43). Chicago: Encyclopaedia Britannica.

ARTICLE in a STANDARD ENCYCLOPAEDIA (Web-site Version)

Islam.(1992). In *Britannica.com*. Retrieved February 9, 2002 from Britannica.com database.

JOURNAL ARTICLE (Paper copy)

Oguisso, T. (1999). Professional nursing in Brazil. *International Nursing Review*, *43*, 81-94.

JOURNAL ARTICLE (from an online database) (for more details, see the APA's official site)

Kavanagh, K., Absalom, K., Beil, W., and Schliessmann, L. (1999). Connecting and becoming culturally competent: A Lakota example. *Advances in Nursing Science, 21,* 9-31. Retrieved March 26, 2001 from ProQuest/Nursing Journals database.

ARTICLE FROM A NEWSPAPER

For job seekers, a toll-free gift of expert advice. (1993, December 12) *New York Times,* p. D1.

ARTICLE FROM A MAGAZINE

Corliss, R. (1993, September 13). Pacific overtures. *Time,* 142, 68-70.

GOVERNMENT DOCUMENT

Commision on Special Education. (1993) *Our future, our children: planning for the next generation* (93-094-P). Washington, DC: Government Printing Office.

PUBLISHED CONFERENCE PROCEEDINGS

Murray, L. (Ed). (2001). *Endless searching: New horizons in search engine technology. Proceedings of the Search Engine Technology Conference, University of Main. Journal of the Internet, 40*(suppl.), 1-402.

JOURNAL ARTICLE (*Online*, on a website) *(for more details, see the APA's official site)*

Outbreak news. (2001, February 23). *Weekly Epidemiological Record, 76,* 57-64. Retrieved February 28, 2001 from http://www.who.int/wer/pdf/2001/wer7608.pdf

MAGAZINE ARTICLE (Paper copy)

Ulrich, T. (1997, September 22). Linking an Amish hereditary disease with cerebral palsy, a pediatrician challenges a dark inheritance. *Time, 150,* 30-33.

MAGAZINE ARTICLE (From an online database)

Ulrich, T. (1997, September 22). Linking an Amish hereditary disease with cerebral palsy, a pediatrician challenges a dark inheritance. *Time, 150,* 30-33. Retrieved March 1, 2001 from InfoTrac/Expanded Academic ASAP database.

NEWSPAPER ARTICLE (Paper copy)

Padilla, H. (2000, June 6). Hugo prohibits custom animal slaughter; the vote will officially close a Hmong slaughterhouse, where animals were sacrificed for religious reasons. *Star Tribune (Minneapolis, MN)*, p. 1B.

NEWSPAPER ARTICLE (From an online database)

Padilla, H. (2000, June 6). Hugo prohibits custom animal slaughter; the vote will officially close a Hmong slaughterhouse, where animals were sacrificed for religious reasons. *Star Tribune (Minneapolis, MN)*, p. 1B. Retrieved February 28, 2001 from Lexis-Nexis Universe/General News database.

PAMPHLET/BROCHURE (Cite like a book but add [Brochure] as shown)

Research and Training Center on Independent Living. (1993). *Guidelines for reporting and writing about people with disabilities* (4th ed.) [Brochure]. Lawrence, KS: Author.

ERIC DOCUMENT

Fredrickson, M. (2000). *Parent/child communication in migrant communities*. Miami, FL: Annual Meeting of the Speech Communication Association. (ERIC Document Reproduction Service No. ED 377 236).

DISSERTATION

If you obtain an actual dissertation (not just its abstract), in print or on microform, check the *Publication Manual of the APA* for complete directions on citing it properly.

DISSERTATION (Abstract only, obtained on CINAHL)

Crow, G. K. (1988). *Toward a theory of therapeutic syncretism: The Southeast Asian experience: A study of the Cambodians' use of traditional and cosmopolitan health systems*.(Doctoral dissertation, University of Utah, 1988).Abstract retrieved March 19, 2001 from CINAHL database.

DISSERTATION (Abstract only, obtained from DAI on First Search)

Crow, G. K. (1988). *Toward a theory of therapeutic syncretism: The Southeast Asian experience: A study of the Cambodians' use of traditional and cosmopolitan health systems* (Doctoral dissertation, University of

Utah, 1988). *Dissertation Abstracts International, 49*(08B), 3101. Abstract retrieved March 19, 2001 from First Search/Dissertation Abstracts International database.

WEBSITE (NOT from an online database) (for more details, see the APA's official site)

The Amish, the Mennonites, and the Plain People. (n.d.). Retrieved May 30, 2000 from Pennsylvania Dutch Country Welcome Center Website: http://www.800padutch.com/amish.shtml

ORGANIZATION AS AUTHOR

Use the full name of the group or corporation for the author's name. Well known abbreviations may be used in subsequent references.

First mention of the reference: (American Medical Association, 2002) Subsequent mention: (AMA, 2002).

INTERVIEWS, E-MAILS, PHONE CONVERSATIONS, etc.

"Because they do not provide recoverable data, personal communications are not included in the reference list. Cite personal communications in text only. Give the initials as well as the surname of the communicator, and provide as exact a date as possible." (*APA Manual*, section 3.102) Example: I. M. Certain (personal communication, April 1, 2000).

PRESENTATIONS, SPEECHES, POSTER SESSIONS, etc.

Like the example above, if they do not provide "recoverable data," these would not be included in the reference list and would be cited in the text only. If, however, something tangible exists (e.g. handouts of PowerPoint slides, an abstract in a conference program, etc.), it might be citable. See the *APA Manual*, section 4.16 D and F. Here is an example of a poster session:

Worral, P. S. and Levin, R. (2004, June). *Developing a statewide research agenda.* Poster session presented at the biannual meeting of the American Nurses Association, Minneapolis, MN.

Since they ask, I have suggested to students who wish to cite a presentation *unofficially*, for an *undergraduate paper*, that they could cite it like this:

Twohy, K. (2004, January 15). Testimony given at Health, Human Services and Corrections Budget Division, St. Cloud, Minnesota.

GOVERNMENT DOCUMENT See How to Cite Government Documents

5.4.3 MODERN LANGUAGE ASSOCIATION

List of Works Cited (Print Materials)

Books, journals, magazines, and newspapers are identified by underlining the title. Article or chapter titles are identified by "quotation marks." "Works Cited" is the heading in the MLA style. Begin each entry flush with the left margin. If an entry runs more than one line, indent the following entry lines 5 spaces. Double space each entry.

Book by One Author

Rattenbury, Ken. Duke Ellington, Jazz Composer. New Haven: Yale UP, 1990.

Book by Two or more Authors

Jakobson, Roman, and Linda R. Waugh. The Sound Shape of Language. Bloomington: Indiana UP, 1975.

An Anthology or Compilation

Frye, Northrop, ed. Sound and Poetry. New York: Columbia UP, 1957.

Work in an Anthology

Allende, Isabel. "Toad's Mouth." Trans. Margaret Sayers Peden. A Hammock beneath the Mangoes: Stories from Latin America. Ed. Thomas Colchie. New York: Plume, 1992. 83-88.

Article from a Magazine

Bazell, Robert. "Science and Society: Growth Industry." New Republic 15 Mar. 1993: 13-14.

Article from a Scholarly Journal

Scotto, Peter. "Censorship, Reading, and Interpretation: A Case Study from the Soviet Union." PMLA 109 (1994): 61-70.

Article from a Newspaper

Feder, Barnaby J. "For Job Seekers, a Toll-Free Gift of Expert Advice." New York Times 30 Dec. 1993, late ed.: D1+.

Government Publication

United States. Congress. Senate. Subcommittee on Constitutional Amendments. Hearings on the "Equal Rights Amendment". 91st Cong., 2nd sess. S. Res. 61. Washington: GPO, 1970.

Articles from an Online Periodical

- Author's name (if given)
- "Title of work" (if any) in quotation marks
- Name of periodical (underlined)
- Volume number, issue number, or other identifying number
- Year of publication
- Range or total number of pages or paragraphs (if available)
- Title of database (underlined)

Scholarly journals available online independently or as part of an archival database of journals (e.g. JSTOR, PCI, Project Muse) provide the following additional information:

Date of access and <URL>

Maynard, W. Barksdale. "Thoreau's House at Walden." Art Bulletin 81.2 (1999): 303-25. JSTOR. 19 Nov. 2002 < http://www.JSTOR.org>.

Bueno, Eva Paulino. "Carolina Maria De Jesus in the Context of Testimonios: Race, Sexuality, and Exclusion." Criticism 41. 2 (1999): 257. Infotrac Expanded Academic ASAP, Gale. 22 Sept. 2000 <http://web4.infotrac.galegroup.com/itw/infomark/>.

Online Reference Database, Scholarly Project, Professional, Personal Site

- Author's name (if given)
- Title of project (underlined)
- Name of editor (if given)

Electronic publication information, including version number, date of electronic publication or last update, and name of sponsoring institution date of access and <URL>

Article in a Reference Database

"Colour" Encyclopaedia Britannica Online. Version 99.1 1999. Encyclopaedia Britannica. 22 December 1999 <http://www.eb.com:180/bol/topic?eu= 117710&sctn=26>.

Scholarly Project

Dickens Project. Ed. Jon Michael Varese. 1999. University of

California, Santa Cruz. 22 December 1999 <http://humwww.ucsc.edu/dickens>.

Professional Site

McHenry Library Instructional Services. Deborah A. Murphy. 20 December 1999. University of California, Santa Cruz . 22 December 1999 <http://library.ucsc.edu/ref/instruction>.

Personal Site

Cayute, Ima. Home page. 10 August 1997 <http://www.cayute.ulib.ca>.

Online Government Publication

United States. Dept. of Justice. Office of Juvenile Justice and Delinquency Prevention. Juvenile Crime. by Henry Smith. Dec. 2001. 29 June 2003 <http://www.ncjrs.org/pdfiles1/191031.pdf>.

Online Book

Author's name (If editor, translator, etc., cite name followed by appropriate abbreviation.)

- ☆ Title of work (underlined)
- ☆ Name of editor, etc. (if relevant)
- ☆ Publication information
- ☆ Date of access and <URL>

Dos Passos, John. One Man's Initiation: 1917; A Novel. Ithaca: Cornell University Press, 1969. 1 January 1999. Internet Modern History Sourcebook. 22 December 1999 <http://eldred.ne.mediaone.net/wwone/initiation.html>.

Article in an Pnline Periodical

- ☆ Author's name (if given)
- ☆ "Title of work" (if any) in quotation marks
- ☆ Name of periodical (underlined)
- ☆ Volume number, issue number, or other identifying number
- ☆ Date of publication
- ☆ Range or total number of pages or paragraphs
- ☆ Date of access and <URL>

Article in Online Journal

Carranza, L.E. "Le Corbusier and the Problems of Representation." Journal of Architectural Education 48.2 (1994). 22 September 1997 <http://wwwmitpress.mit.edu/jrnls-catalog/arch-ed-abstracts/File:jae48- 2.html>.

Article in Online Newspaper

Ferriss, Susan. "Latino Rock - Hot Like a 'Volcano': Mission District Label 1st to Focus on Trend." San Francisco Examiner 16 July 1995. 23 Sept. 1997 <http://www.examiner.com>.

Article in Online Magazine

Mindiola, Jim. "Selena and Me: A Virtual Chicano's Journey of Discovery." Frontera 2.1(1997).17Sept.1997<http://www.mercado.com/frontera/current/Selena/index.htm>.

Publication on CD-ROM, Disk, or Magnetic Tape

- Author's name (If editor, translator, etc., cite name followed by appropriate abbreviation.)
- Title of publication (underlined)
- Name or editor, etc. (if relevant)
- Publication medium (CD-ROM, etc.)
- Edition, release or version (if relevent)
- Place of publication
- Name of publisher
- Date of publication

Singh, Susheela. "Early Marriage Among Women in Developing Countries." International Family Planning Perspectives 22.4 (1996): 148+. Contemporary Women's Issues. CD-ROM. RDS, Inc. 1992-present.

5.4.4 COMPARISON OF APA and MLA CITATIONS

Book with One Author

APA: Sagan, C. (1980). *Cosmos*. New York: Random House.

MLA: Sagan, Carl. *Cosmos*. New York: Random House. 1980.

Book with Two Authors

APA: Calfee, R. C., and Valencia, R. R. (1991). *APA guide to preparing manuscripts for journal publication*. Washington, DC: American Psychological Association.

MLA: Bohlman, Herbert M., and Mary Jane Dundas. *The Legal, Ethical and International Environment of Business*. 5th ed. Cincinnati, OH: West, 2002.

Edited Book

APA: O'Neil, J. M., and Egan, J. (1992). Men's and women's gender role journeys: Metaphor for healing, transition, and transformation. In B. R. Wainrib (Ed.), *Gender issues across the life cycle* (pp. 107-123). New York: Springer.

MLA: Swanson, Gunnar. "Graphic Design Education as a Liberal Art: Design and Knowledge in the University and The 'Real World.'" *The Education of a Graphic Designer*. Ed. Steven Heller. New York: Allworth Press, 1998. 13-24.

Journal Article

If there are more than six authors, list the first six and then use: *et al.*

APA: Hlastala, S. A. Frank, E. Kowalski, J. Sherrill, J. T. Tu, X. M. Anderson, B. Kupfer, D. J. (2000). Stressful life events, bipolar disorder, and the "kindling model. *Journal of abnormal psychology*, 109(4):777 - 86.

MLA: Nielsen, Laura Beth. "Subtle, Pervasive, Harmful: Racist and Sexist Remarks in Public as Hate Speech." *Journal of Social Issues* 58.2 (2002): 265.

Article from an Online Journal

APA: Monroe, S. Harkness, K. (2005). Life Stress, the "Kindling" Hypothesis, and the Recurrence of Depression: Considerations From a Life Stress Perspective. *Psychological Review*, 112 (2). 417 – 445. Retrieved from: http://psyc.queensu.ca/~harkness/documents/PR_Kindling_Paper.pdf

MLA: Nielsen, Laura Beth. "Subtle, Pervasive, Harmful: Racist and Sexist Remarks in Public as Hate Speech." Journal of Social Issues 58.2 (2002), 265-280. 7 June 2003. <http://www.blackwell-synergy.com/doi/abs/10.1111/1540-4560.00260>.

Reference and further Reading

American Psychological Association Style Manual. http://www.apastyle.org

University of Maryland University College – Library services. http://www.umuc.edu/library/guides/apa.shtml

APA: available at http://en.wikipedia.org/wiki/APA_style (Accessed on 2nd June, 2011)

Cooper, H. M. (1988), "The structure of knowledge synthesis". In *Knowledge in Society*, Vol. 1, pp. 104-126.

Harvard System: http://libweb.anglia.ac.uk/referencing/harvard.htm (Accessed on 5th June, 2011).

MLA: available at http://honolulu.hawaii.edu/library/mlahcc.html (Accessed on 2nd June, 2011).

Chapter 6

CD-ROM Databases and Online Catalogues

6.1 Information Storage Media

Due to the enormous growth of information as a result of research and development, more and more data is needed to be stored and retrieved. This has resulted in development of various technologies to meet the information storage and retrieval. These storage technologies can be divided into Magnetic storage and Optical Storage.

6.1.1 Magnetic Storage

With magnetic storage, the computer stores data on disks and tapes by magnetizing selected particles of an oxide-based surface coating. The particles retain their magnetic orientation until that orientation is changed, thereby making disks and tape fairly permanent but modifiable storage media. Users can intentionally change or erase files stored on magnetic media. Data stored on magnetic media can also be unintentionally altered. Magnetic media can be disrupted by magnetic fields and gradually lose their magnetic charge and lose data. The reliable life span of data stored on magnetic media is about three years and recommend that users refresh data every two years by recopying it. It is important to realize that data stored on magnetic media is subject to device and media failures, which make the data unusable. Magnetic storage and retrieval systems include: flexible disk, hard disk, and tape.

6.1.2 Optical Storage

Optical media is the most preferred storing device in the flourishing information era for storing large amount of data which makes use of beams of laser light. Therefore, most common optical storage is read only memory (ROM) but some types of optical storage media allow user to read, write, erase, and modify files. Magneto optical drives merge magnetic and optical technologies. So users can read, write, erase, and modify files, as on a hard disk drive, but they offer very large storage capacity and reliable long-term storage. Optical storage and retrieval systems include: photo CD, videodisk. Compact Disc Read Only Memory (CD-ROM), Write Once Read Many disk (WORM disk), Erasable Optical Storage disk (EOS disk), CD-Recordable (CD-R), CD-Interactive (CD-I), and Digital Versatile Disk (DVD).

Introduced in 1997, the next generation of optical storage technology is the DVD, which stands for Digital Video Disc. The primary advantage of DVD is the tremendous jump in storage capacity from the CD-ROMs 650MB to 17GB even though the discs are the same size. DVD discs can contain from two to eight hours of high-quality digital video that is ideally suited for movies. They can support up to eight tracks of digital audio besides facilitates to listen to commentary from actors and directors or even a foreign language translation and DVD discs are exceptionally durable. For the sharing of information over CD jukeboxes to DVD jukebox with discs flipping capability under networked environ, Network Attached Storage (NAS) has been quite popularly used for accessing information over networks. As a result of these new developments in the library industry include network attached storage (NAS), more advanced library controllers, and most importantly, new tape formats are being used.

CD-ROM

CD-ROM is an abbreviation of Compact Disc Read-Only Memory used for information and retrieval of information accessed by a computer. Basically, CD-ROM format was originally designed for music storage and playback, but later, the format adapted to store any form of binary data which includes audio, video, data, and graphs. It is popularly used to distribute computer software, including games and multimedia applications, though any data can be stored of 650 to 750 MB capacity limit.

CD-ROM discs are made from a 1.2 mm thick disc of polycarbonate plastic, with a thin layer of aluminum to make a reflective surface. The most common size of CD-ROM disc is 120 mm in diameter, though the smaller Mini CD standard with an 80 mm diameter, as well as numerous non-standard sizes and shapes. A CD-ROM sector contains 2352 bytes, divided into 98 24-byte frames. The CD-ROM is, in essence, a data disk, which cannot rely on error concealment, and therefore requires a higher reliability of the retrieved data. A standard 74 min CD contains 333,000 sectors and each sector is 2352 bytes, and contains 2048 bytes of PC (MODE1) Data, 2336 bytes of PSX/VCD (MODE2) Data or 2352 bytes of AUDIO.

CD-ROM is a new storage medium that can serve as a quick, economical source of information for students, researchers, writers, and professionals in many fields. This digest will address some commonly asked questions that beginning or novice users may have about CD-ROM database services.

DVD

DVD stands for Digital Video Disc, is an optical disc storage media format used for data storage and retrieval including movies with high video and sound quality. DVDs resemble compact discs as their physical dimensions are the same (120 mm (4.72 inches) or occasionally 80 mm (3.15 inches) in diameter) but they are encoded in a different format and at a much higher density. The official DVD specification is maintained by the DVD Forum.

In the early 1990s two high-density optical storage standards were being developed: one was the Multimedia Compact Disc (MMCD), backed by Philips and Sony, and the other was the Super Density disc (SD), supported by Toshiba, Time-Warner, Matsushita Electric, Hitachi, Mitsubishi Electric, Pioneer, Thomson, and JVC. The first DVD players and discs were available in November 1996 in Japan, March 1997 in the United States, 1998 in Europe and in 1999 in Australia. The first pressed DVD release was the film Twister in 1996. The film had the first test for 2.1 surround sound. The first titles released in the U.S., on March 19, 1997, by Lumivision, authored by AIX Entertainment, were IMAX adaptations.

There has been lot of transformation in information storage media especially for research abstract databases which were brought in CD-ROM format are now made available in DVD format especially Biological Abstracts. The CD-ROMs and DVDs are more flexible and less prone to damage for storing large amount of information and facilitates easy retrieval of information at the finger tips.

Pen Drives/USB Flash Drives

USB flash drives are memory data storage devices integrated with a USB interface and are typically small, lightweight, removable and rewritable storage devices looks like small pen. The memory capacity typically ranges from megabytes up to 64 gigabytes limited only by current flash memory densities. The flash drive was first invented in 1998 by Dov Moran, President and CEO of M-Systems Flash Pioneers (Israel).

USB flash drives have several advantages over other portable storage devices, particularly the floppy disk and CD-ROM devices as they are generally faster, hold more data, handy, very portable and are considered more reliable due to their lack of moving parts than floppy disks. Flash drives are nearly impervious to the scratches and dust that were problematic for previous forms of portable storage, such as compact discs and floppy disks, and their durable solid-state design means they often survive casual abuse. This makes them ideal for transporting personal data or work files from one location to another, such as from home to school or office or for carrying around personal data that the user typically wants to access in a variety of places. The near-ubiquity of USB support on modern computers means that such a drive will work in most places. Flash drives are also a relatively dense form of storage, where even the cheapest will store dozens of floppy disks worth of data. Some can hold more data than a CD-ROM.

Zip Drives

The Zip drives just like CD-Drive a medium-capacity removable disk storage system, introduced by Iomega in late 1994. It is a small, portable disk drive used primarily for backing up and archiving personal computer files. Originally it had a capacity of 100 MB, but later versions increased this to first 250 MB and then 750 MB. The format became the most popular of the super-floppy type products but never reached the status of a quasi-standard to replace the 3.5-

inch floppy disk. The Zip brand was also used for internal and external CD writers known as Zip-650 or Zip-CD. It was short lived in the computer market although more reliable due to latest storage technologies which has been superseded by flash-drive systems as well as rewritable CDs and DVDs, and is fading in popularity.

CD-NAS Server

Network Attached Storage (NAS) systems are networked appliances which contain one or more hard drives, often arranged into logical, redundant storage containers or RAID arrays. Network-attached storage removes the responsibility of file serving from other servers on the network. CD/DVD server will use the hard drive to make an image copy of each CD/DVD to share on the network. The capacity of these CD NAS server runs in terabytes and consolidates multiple CD/DVD towers into a single caching server and save rack or floor space. Reduce collocation costs. No longer have to hand out expensive CD/DVDs to users but these CD/DVDs image is created on the server and make them secure and accessible on the network.

Ex: CD NAS Server - 2084 MB memory, DVD writer drive, 500 GB SATA Hard Disk Drive (4 TB and more).

CD-ROM Databases

CD-ROM is a form of optical disk or laserdisc technology that is similar to the popular digital audio compact disk, or CD. As their name implies, CDs are written to and read by the concentrated light beam of a laser. The laser creates tiny pits, representing bits of digitized information, on the plastic surface of the disk. An optical disk can contain information in any form, including audio, video, text, graphics, or a combination. Unlike magnetic media (audio and videotapes, floppy and hard computer disks), optical disks are almost error-free and indestructible.

CD-ROM is a compact disk with read-only memory: information stored on it cannot be changed. The most conspicuous advantage of CD-ROM is its large storage capacity. One disk with 550 megabyte capacity can store 220,000 pages of text, or the equivalent of about 1,500 floppy disks. Used with a microcomputer, CD-ROM greatly expands the microcomputer's ability to deliver information in an interactive environment. CD-ROM databases can be accessed directly by users, thus freeing them from the necessity of consulting (and paying) an expert to do online mainframe searches. Information from many CD-ROM databases can be downloaded to floppy disk for later use with a word processor or other software, or printed on paper.

CD-ROM does have several disadvantages. Its greatest drawback is that information cannot be added or erased by the user. And CD-ROM still does not have the storage capacity to handle full-text documents in very large databases: many are indexes containing citations with abstracts. A number of databases are updated monthly or quarterly, but for current information such as news, this may not be sufficient. And while CD-ROM is capable of storing mixed media, most publishers offer text because text requires the least storage space. Full-motion video is not yet economical. Finally, the hardware does not allow a full range of flexibility and compatibility for those who wish to use more than one CD-ROM product.

Educational information particularly indexing and abstracting sources are available in CD-ROM format including reference sources and full text information sources. Some of the popular abstracting databases available in CD-ROM format are:

Database	*Period*	*Publishers*
Math-Science	1980+	Silver Platter, USA
Biological Abstracts	1992+	Silver Platter, USA
Biotechnology Abstracts	1982+	Silver Platter, USA
Sociological Abstracts	1974+	Silver Platter, USA
Econ-Lit	1969+	Silver Platter, USA
Psych-Info	1887+	Silver Platter, USA
Cross Culture	Vol. 1-5	Silver Platter, USA
Georef	1785+	Silver Platter, USA
Eric	1966+	Silver Platter, USA
LISA	1969+	CSA
Dissertation Abstracts International	1861+	UMI, U.K
ABI/Inform	1989+	UMI, U.K
INSPEC	1989+	I.E.E.E
CABSAC (South Asian)	1973+	Informatics India Pvt. Ltd.
IBID	1993+	Informatics India Pvt. Ltd.

Database	Period	Publishers
Supreme Court Online	1950+	Eastern Book Co., India
VET CD	1973+	CABI Publishing
MEDLARS	1971	National Library of Medicine
AGRICOLOA (**AGRIC**ultural **O**n**L**ine **A**ccess)	1970+	National Agricultural Library and the research of the U.S. Department of Agriculture (USDA)
AGRIS (International System for Agricultural Science and Technology)	1975+	FAO, http://agris.fao.org
FSTA (Food Science and Technology Abstracts)	1969 +	International Food Information Service (IFIS)

CD-ROM Databases (Bibliographic): The CD-ROM databases which are available in CD-Rom and now with the tremendous impact of information technology is made available on the Internet. The details of online cum CD-ROM databases are briefed as under:

Today, a large number of companies around the world are publishing scientific data, bibliographic and full text on CD-ROMs. Silver Platter publishes the largest number of CD-ROM databases in the field of agrobiological sciences and other branches of Science and technology, medicine, social sciences and humanities. Some of the important databases on CD-ROMs published in the field of agriculture and allied sciences are mentioned here:

Biosis Databases on CD-ROM available are:

- ☆ Biological Abstracts on CD (1985)
- ☆ Biological Abstracts /RRM on CD (1989)
- ☆ Zoological Record on CD (1985)
- ☆ Biosis Gen Ref on CD (1985)
- ☆ Foods Intelligence on CD (1985)
- ☆ Toxline plus on CD (1985)

Biological Abstracts (BA) on CD-ROM

Biological Abstracts on CD is published since 1985 and presents the most comprehensive life science journal literature, including agriculture, biochemistry, biotechnology, botany, ecology, environment, microbiology, neurology, Pharmacology and public health and monitoring 6,500 journals in the life science discipline. In 19 CDs it contains about 5 million records 3,60,000 records are added annually with quarterly updates.

Biological Abstracts (BA)/RRM on CD ROM

Similar to Biological Abstracts (Reviews, Reports, and Meetings)/RRM contains literature on life sciences from reports, reviews, meetings literature, books, patents, etc. The database contains about 16,00,000 records since 1989 with annual additions of 2,16,000 records comprising of Review articles (16,500) meeting literature (1,40,000) books (27,500) and patents (12,000).

Zoological Record on CD-ROM

It provides the most comprehensive coverage of world wide zoological literature. 72,000 records are added annually monitoring over 6,500 internationals, annual reviews, monographs, proceedings literature, books and reports for inclusion in Biosis. All major branches of zoology are represented including animal and insect behavior, ecology, evolution, habitat, nutrition, parasitology, reproduction, zoogeography, animal and dairy science, etc. It contains 12,30,000 bibliographic records since 1985.

Biosis Gen Ref on CD-ROM

It contains over one million bibliographical references with abstracts since 1985. It is the single reference source for multi-disciplinary genetics information. It covers plant, animal human and micro organism genetics. The compact disc offers the widest collection of scientific findings, over 75,000 gene sequence numbers from 1985 to date from Gene Bank, EMBL and DDBJ repositories. About 1,00,000 abstracts are added annually on the subjects like biology, biotechnology, DNA Genetics, government regulations, medicine and health sciences, industry news and marketing.

Foods Intelligence on CD-ROM

The CD contains about 4,50,000 abstracts from 1985 out of Biosis database. It provides the most comprehensive information on food industry and useful for scientists, research scholars, food technologists and business community. It covers subjects like aquaculture, genetic engineering nutrition and food preparation, food packaging, labeling, new product launches and government regulations.

Toxline Plus on CD

It contains about 1.4 million bibliographic records since 1985 to date out of Biosis and other sources and provides information on chemical substance reactions, drugs, environment pollution, hazardous and waste material, health and safety, toxicology, etc.

CAB International CDs

CAB International has published its database on CD-ROMs in 5 volumes since 1973 to date. They contain in all about 3 million records with abstracts on different aspects of agriculture, like agronomy, botany, horticulture, fertilizers, entomology, ecology and environment, economics, animal and dairy science and aquaculture.

CABI also has issued speciality database CD-ROM s under its spectrum Series just like it's by – product commodity based speciality abstracts, namely.

- ☆ **Ag Econ CD:** It offers a comprehensive coverage of literature on agricultural economics since 1973. It contains 2,40,000 abstracts on socio-economic aspects of agriculture, forestry and rural development including subjects like agricultural economics, policy and planning, food industry, marketing and distribution, trade and finance, etc.
- ☆ **CAB Pest CD:** Subjects covered are entomology, plant pathology, nematology, weed science, agricultural chemicals, pesticides and environment.
- ☆ **Crop CD:** Covers subjects like agronomy, botany, biochemistry, crop physiology, crop production, farming systems, cereals, legumes, oilseeds, root crops, fiber, sugarcane, tobacco, etc.
- ☆ **E-CD- CD-ROM** on environmental quality covers topic like soil erosion and control, biodegradation, bioremediation, environmental issues like deforestation, biological treatment of wastes, impact of tourism on the environment and various other socio-economic aspects of agriculture, forestry, food and rural development. The CD contains over 5, 25,000 references since 1973 to the present.
- ☆ **HORT CD:** This CD covers horticultural literature on the subjects like tree fruits, and nuts, vegetables, ornamental plants, minor industrial crops, along with information on

their cultivation, propagation, planting, soils and fertilizer, nutrition, crop management, plant breeding and genetics, post harvest technology and fruit industry, etc. Hort CD contains 4.5 lakhs records with abstracts since 1973.

- ☆ **Plant Gene CD:** Plant Gene CD since 1973 to date contains about 4, 60,000 bibliographic references with abstracts on agricultural, horticultural, plantation and forestry crops. The subject as pests, plant breeding, cytogenetics and taxonomy, intellectual property rights and other crops like forest trees, ornamental plants and edible fungi have been covered.
- ☆ **Soil CD:** This CD covers literature on soil science and contains over 3,60,000 abstracts since 1973 to date. It provides a comprehensive coverage of soils, fertilizers and water management, irrigation, agricultural meteorology, crop management, environment and pollution, land, soils and nutrients and agronomic aspects.
- ☆ **Tree CD:** Tree CD contains bibliographic citations and abstracts published in Forestry Abstracts from its first volume (published in 1939) to the present day. It also covers abstracts published in Forest Products Abstracts and Agro forestry Abstracts. The Tree CD offers over 3, 60,000 records on agriculture, forestry, environment, tree pests, etc.
- ☆ **Vet CD:** On veterinary sciences, the Vet CD contains about 5, 75,000 bibliographic records since 1973 to present. Subjects covered into the Vet CD include animal science and animals, zoology and Veterinary science and as such it deals with aspects of arthropod, helminthes, protozoa, animal diseases, wild fish, shellfish, zoo animals, wild animals, pets and farm animals.

AGRICOLA on CD-ROM

Agricola (NAL, USA) on CD ROMs since 1970 contains 3.3 million bibliographic references with abstracts on agriculture and allied subjects *viz.*, agronomy, plant breeding, soils and fertilizers, water, nutrition, pesticides, botany, genetics, horticulture, forestry, animal, veterinary and dairy sciences, entomology, aquaculture, environment and natural resources. The data consist of journal articles, monographs, theses, technical reports, patents etc. in the field.

Dissertation Abstracts International (DIA)

Dissertation Abstracts International from the University Microfilms International, (Michigan, USA) is a monthly abstracts service in print form in two series –(a) Humanities and social sciences, (b) Sciences and Engineering , Now, the Dissertation Abstracts on CD incorporates Dissertations, and comprehensive dissertation Index. DAI contains 12, 00,000 citations since 1861 on biotechnology, chemistry, maths, medicine, pharmaceuticals, veterinary science and zoology etc. along with economics, education, psychology, etc.

Food and Human Nutrition on CD-ROM

A database from AGRIS coordinating Group of FAO offers bibliographic literature on agriculture, food and nutrition, health sciences, etc. It contains 311,000 records and about 25,000 records are added annually. CD is updated semi-annually.

Food Science and Technology Abs tracts (FSTA)

FSTA from International Food Information Service (IFIS) is a comprehensive database which covers various aspects of food science, food products and food processing including biotechnology, economics, dairy science, food manufacturing, food microbiology, food legislation and packaging of processed food products. FSTA C contains about 5, 00,000 bibliographic records since 1969 to date, scanned from 2000 core scientific journals in the field of Food Science and Technology.

Chemical Abstracts on CD

The Chemical Abstracts (CA) since 1907 has been published from the American Chemical Society (Colombia) as weekly service along with its cumulative indexes. Semi annual, decimal and 5 yearly indexes. CA after a long journey of 87 years published its 15 millionth abstract in volume 120 (no.12) on March 7, 1994. Its each weekly issue appends (i) author, (ii) chemical substance and (iii) formula indexes. Now the Chemical Abstracts are available on CD-ROMs.

Science Citation Index (SCI)

Institute for Scientific Information (Philadelphia) publishes Science Citation Index in 3 parts (i) Citation Index (ii) Subject Permuterm Index and (iii) Source Index along with Journal Citation

Reports and Index of Scientific and Technical Proceedings. SCI database covers citation literature from over 3300 core journals. The SCI on CD-ROM contains citations from 1980 on all applied and theoretical sciences including agrobiological sciences.

Current Contents on CD-ROM

The fastest Current Awareness Service (CAS) "Current Contents" (CC) issued in different series, *viz.*, (i) CC: Agriculture, Biology and Environmental Sciences (ii) CC: Life Sciences, (iii) CC: Social and Behavioural Sciences etc. Apart from its Diskette edition it is available on CD-ROM presents an entire year's worth of current contents published data and thus provides the facility of browsing or searching 52 continuous weeks of information at a time. Thus, it facilitates the data/ information search on a computer network.

CD-ROM Databases (Full Text)

Similar to abstracts on CD-ROMs now a large number of scientific journals with full text articles are being published on CD ROMs around the world. Many leading publishers like Blackwell Scientific Publishers, UK, Kluwer Academic Publishers and Elsevier Science, Netherlands, Springer-Verlag, Germany, Academic Press Journals, UK, Annual Reviews Inc, USA, have created full text databases of their journals in electronic form. These journals are also available on Internet in electronic form. These journals are also available on Internet. Some other magazines like nature, Science, Journal of Extension are available on Internet. It seems that in future more and more scientific journals will be available on CD-ROMs. Some important journals on CD-ROMs are mentioned here.

- ☆ Journals of Virology
- ☆ Journal of Cell Science
- ☆ Journal of Experimental Biology

ADONIS (1991-1996)

Provides images of Full Text articles appearing in 798 Biomedical Journals published by 80 European and North American Publishers.

- ☆ Business Periodicals On disc (BPO)
- ☆ (Global Edition) (1987-2002)

- ☆ Contains abstracts of articles from more than 800??/2218 management and business journals.
- ☆ Contains full text of articles from more than 480 of these journals.

AHEAD: Asian Health, Environmental and Allied Databases (1995-)

Contains full-text and bibliographic databases related to water management, recycling of waste water, hygiene education and community participation. "Wealth Asia", contains the entire Medicinal and Aromatic Plants bibliographic database mentioned above and a full-text database of Indian plant, animal and mineral resources, based on the well known "Wealth of India" encyclopaedic book series.

Chemical Abstract on CD (1996-)

Covers scientific disciplines including biomedical sciences, chemistry, engineering, material science, agricultural science, etc. Provides journal article references (with abstracts) from nearly 9500 major scientific journals worldwide and patent and patent family references from 50 active patent issuing authorities around the world. Offers value-added content from journals and patents

Current Contents (2000-2004) (Now: Online 1998+)

ABES, ECT, LS, PCES

ExtraMED Biomedical Journals Library (1994-1996)

Contains full text, as page images, of the papers from over best 300 Third World biomedical journals Focuses on journals excluded from international indexes *e.g.* MEDLINE Largest source of full text biomedical literature from developing countries (India, Pakistan, China, Philippines, Hong Kong, Korea, Singapore and others). Covers literature from traditional medicine, tropical medicine etc.

Indian Standards on CD-ROM (Start-2004)

LISA Plus: Library and Information Science Abstracts (1969-; plus Online 1969+)

Provides information on all area of library and information science from 440 periodicals from more than 68 countries and in more than 20 different languages.

Ulrich's Plus: Periodical Directory (1996+)

Provides detailed information of a periodical including publisher, history, subscription, circulation, availability , subject, coverage, etc. covers about 4,26,800 periodicals published world over, searchable on title, country, subject, publisher, keyword, ISSN, CODEN, Dewey Decimal or Library of Congress Class Number, etc.

Science Citation Index (SCI) (1980+)

Provides access to current bibliographic information and cited references, covers approximately 3,500 of the world's leading scientific and technical journals in a broad range of disciplines. Cited reference searching; optional searchable author abstracts; Related Records; author keywords; Keywords Plus; and author names and addresses. Annual SCI-CD's are available from 1980. SCI CD-ROM with Abstracts Edition available from 2006.

US Patents (1990-1994 (Full Text); 1995-2002 (Images)

Provides full text / graphic image of the actual patent including text, drawings, schematics and structures. provides search on: Patent number; Issue date; Application number; Filing date; Priority number; International Class; US class; Inventor; Patent owner (Assignee); and Title / Abstract.

Indian Science Abstracts on CD-ROM

Single source of comprehensive S&T information generated in India. A database of nearly 2 lakhs Indian science abstracts of original research articles short communications, review articles, informative articles, patents, standards and theses covering the period from 1990 onwards. Searchable by keyword, author, corporate author, issue number and year of publication, source journal, and type of document.

National Union Catalogue of Scientific Serials in India (NUCSSI) on CD-ROM

Valuable information tool and provides location information of serials. Covers holdings information of nearly 425 major libraries in India. Updated till 2001 Searchable through various options like journal title, library, city, and subject. Helps in rationalized acquisition of serial in libraries by encouraging resource sharing.

Indian Patents on CD-ROM

Bibliographic database that provides information on more than 52,600 patents granted in India from the year 1975 to 2002. Information about a patent comprises patent title, applicant(s) and inventor(s) names, patent and application numbers, application and publication dates, International Classification Code and country. Database searchable by keywords from title, applicant(s) and inventor(s) names, patent number, application number, application date, publication date, international classification code and subject. Useful to scientists, researchers, patents attorneys and patent offices, libraries of R& D units and business houses.

AGRICOLA, (1970 -)

AGRICultural On-line Access is a machine-readable database of bibliographic records created by the National Agricultural Library and its cooperators. The records describe publications and resources encompassing all aspects of agriculture and allied disciplines, including plant and animal sciences, forestry, entomology, soil and water resources, agricultural economics, agricultural engineering, agricultural products, alternative farming practices, and food and nutrition. Auxiliary subjects that support NAL's Information Center activities, such as agricultural trade and marketing, rural information, and animal welfare, are also included.

- ☆ **AGRIS**, 1975 - August, 2010 (Internet address of the AGRIS–International Information System for the Agricultural Sciences and Technology database) The bibliographic database on the research publications in agriculture and its related fields.
- ☆ **AGRIS Fisheries**, 1975 – 1993

  The bibliographic database on fishery.
- ☆ **AGRIS Food and Human Nutrition**, 1975 – June, 2006

  The bibliographic database on the problems of food and nutrition.
- ☆ **AGRIS Forestry**, 1986 – 1995

  The bibliographic database on forestry.
- ☆ **CARIS**, 1997

  The database contains information on agricultural research projects that have not been finished yet and are being elaborated.

☆ **Veterinary Science Database (Former Title: VETCD),** 1972 –

Veterinary Science Database contains all of the abstracts and citations published in Index Veterinarius and Veterinary Bulletin covers all aspects of veterinary medicine and anthropod, helminth, protozoal and fungal diseases of domestic and wild animals. A majority of records are provided with full, informative abstract.

☆ **AGRICULTURE AND FISHERIES,** 1998

Statistical yearbook of agriculture, forestry and fisheries in the European Union.

☆ **AGRICULTURE and LIFE SCIENCES**

The database contains information from different agricultural reference books and collections of the USA libraries, USDA, and land-grant universities.

☆ **AGRONOMY JOURNAL,** Volumes 1-28 (1907 - 1936)

The database contains articles from the "Agronomy Journal" (volumes 1 - 28) from 1907 to 1936.

☆ **ANNUAL REVIEW OF PHYTOPATHOLOGY** 1986-1995

CD-ROM is special supplement to the Annual Review of Phytopathology, volume 33. It contains full text and images published between 1986 and 1995 and full text and images selected from the following series: Ecology and Systematics, Entomology, Plant Psychology and Plant Molecular Biology, Microbiology, Bioshemistry, Genetics, Cell Biology, Biophysics and Biomolecular Structure.

☆ **CARE** - COMPENDIUM OF ANIMAL RESOURCES

CARE contains Federal legislation and regulations, policies and quidelines of professional scientific societies, bibliographies and full-text articles and monographs. Disc contains 163 documents related to animal care, use and welfare.

☆ **ENCYCLOPAEDIA BRITANNICA [CD]**

The multimedia database is a universal source of knowledge. It contains 72000 records, different pictures, sound records and articles with video or animation.

- ☆ **ENCYCLOPAEDIA BRITANNICA [DVD], 2001, 2002, 2005, 2006, 2008**

  The multimedia database is a universal source of knowledge. It contains 80000 records, different pictures, sound records and articles with video or animation.

- ☆ **INDIASTAT.COM**

  It is a comprehensive statistical information portal that provides recent, exhaustive, authentic socio-economic statistical, political and other country's related information. This database is available online and also on CD-ROM format. It is a cluster of 51 sites including India-specific, Sector specific and State specific sites rendering its dedicated services to the research fraternity from academic, professional and corporate world with authentic and comprehensive compilation of secondary level socio-economic statistical data about India and its states on more than 35 variables.

6.2 Online Public Access Catalogue

The library is a service-oriented institution which facilitates the users with its rich information resources through catalogue. With the advancement of Information and Communication technology, applications of Computer technology with dedicated library software's has enabled the libraries to develop new service known as Online Public Access Catalogue (OPAC) to the users. This reflects the library holdings in machine-readable format providing various searching access points like author, title, call number, Keywords etc.

The development of information technology and library software's in different platforms has enabled the library and information centers to host their bibliographical records on the Internet termed as Web OPAC. The OPAC in the networked environment is confined to the users within a campus, whereas the Web-OPAC extends its identity to the world by putting its resources made available in the bibliographical format.

Some of the major online catalogues in India are discussed below:

6.2.1 AGRICAT@E-GRANTH (http://egranth.ac.in/)

Indian National Agricultural Research System (NARS) has a large collection of Books and articles in agriculture and allied

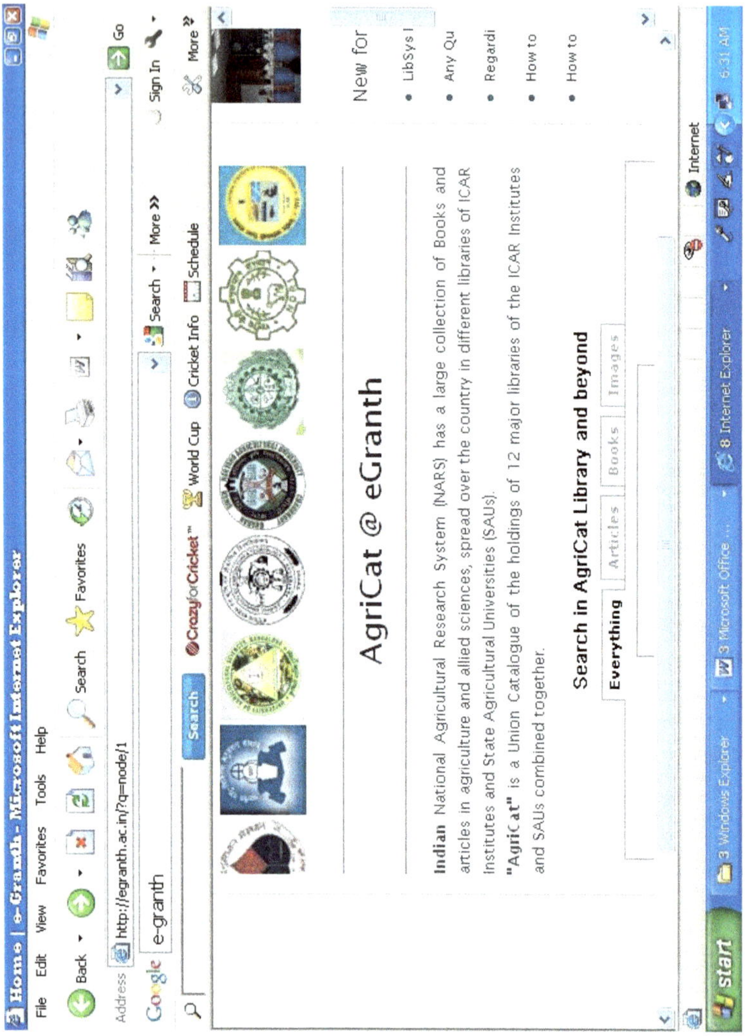
Home | e-Granth - Microsoft Internet Explorer
File Edit View Favorites Tools Help
Back Search Favorites
Address http://egranth.ac.in/?q=node/1
Go
Google e-granth
Search More »
Sign In
Search
CrazyforCricket™ World Cup Cricket Info Schedule
More »
AgriCat @ eGranth
Indian National Agricultural Research System (NARS) has a large collection of Books and articles in agriculture and allied sciences, spread over the country in different libraries of ICAR Institutes and State Agricultural Universities (SAUs).
"AgriCat" is a Union Catalogue of the holdings of 12 major libraries of the ICAR Institutes and SAUs combined together.
Search in AgriCat Library and beyond
Everything
Articles
Books
Images
New for
LibSys I
Any Qu
Regardi
How to
How to
Internet
start
3 Windows Explorer
3 Microsoft Office ...
8 Internet Explorer
6:31 AM

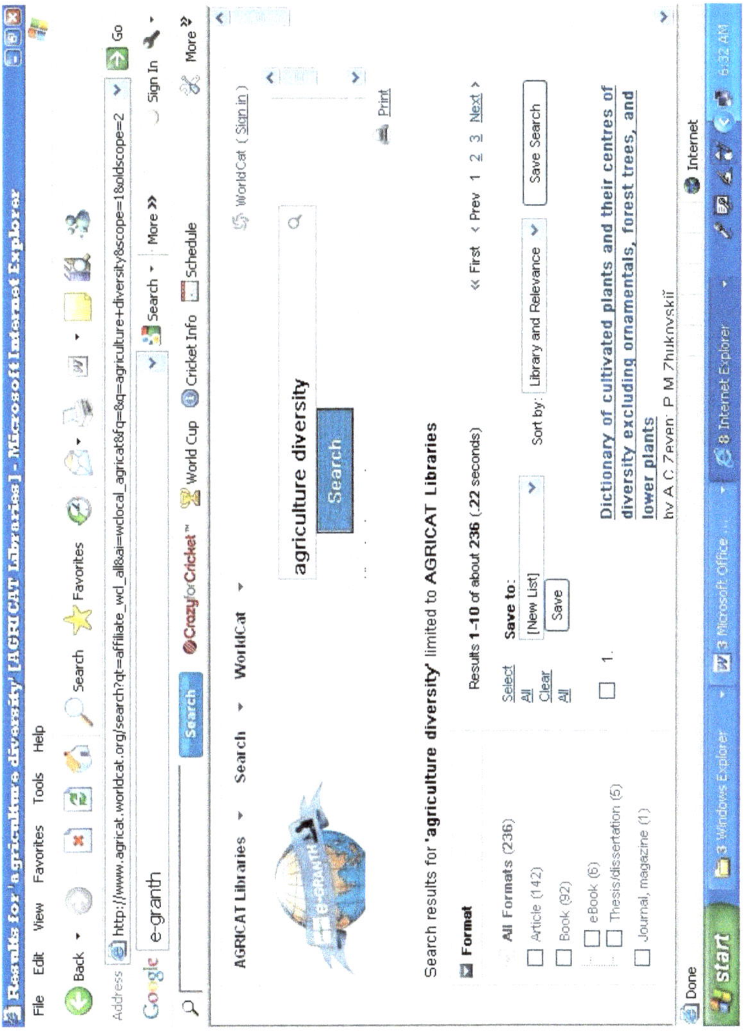
Results for 'agriculture diversity' [AGRICAT Libraries] - Microsoft Internet Explorer
File Edit View Favorites Tools Help
Back Search Favorites
Address http://www.agricat.worldcat.org/search?qt=affiliate_wcl_all&ai=wclocal_agricat&fq=&q=agriculture+diversity&scope=1&oldscope=2
Go
e-granth
Search More »
Sign In
CrazyforCricket World Cup Cricket Info Schedule
More
AGRICAT Libraries Search WorldCat
WorldCat (Sign in)
agriculture diversity
Search
Print
Search results for 'agriculture diversity' limited to AGRICAT Libraries
Format
All Formats (236)
Article (142)
Book (92)
eBook (6)
Thesis/dissertation (5)
Journal, magazine (1)
Results 1-10 of about 236 (.22 seconds)
« First ‹ Prev 1 2 3 Next ›
Select All Clear All
Save to: [New List] Save
Sort by: Library and Relevance
Save Search
1.
Dictionary of cultivated plants and their centres of diversity excluding ornamentals, forest trees, and lower plants
Done
Internet
start
3 Windows Explorer
3 Microsoft Office
8 Internet Explorer
6:32 AM

sciences, spread over the country in different libraries of ICAR Institutes and State Agricultural Universities. **"AgriCat"** is a Union Catalogue of the holdings of 12 major libraries of the ICAR Institutes and SAUs combined together. This union catalogue provides digital access to library resources of 12 different research institutes and agricultural universities which include OPAC, important institutional repositories, rare books and old journals and makes them publically accessible over internet under NARS with Online Computer Library Center (OCLC) partnership.

The main objective of this project is to create Online Public Access Catalog (OPAC) under "Indian Agricultural Research Group Catalogue" of all 12 library resources with Online Computer Library Center (OCLC) partnership; digitize important institutional repositories (limited to IARI, New Delhi; IVRI, Izatnagar; ANGRAU, Hyderabad and UAS, Bangalore) including rare books and old journals and make them open access under NARS and thereby strengthen capacity building for library and information management system.

6.2.2 Worldcat (http://www.worldcat.org/)

WorldCat is the world's largest network of library content and services. WorldCat libraries are dedicated to providing access to their resources on the Web, where most people start their search for information. It facilitates searching of popular books, music CDs and videos and other physical items. The catalogue enables to search many libraries at once for an item and then locate it in a library nearby and connects to the collections and services of more than 10,000 libraries worldwide.

6.2.3 KrishiPrabha - Database of Indian Agricultural Doctoral Dissertations (http://202.141.47.8:8080/equestthesis/)

KrishiPrabha is a full-text online database of Indian Agricultural Doctoral Dissertations submitted by research scholars to the 45 State/ Deemed Agricultural Universities during the period from 1.1.2000 to 31.12.2007. This database, listing about 7500 Doctoral Dissertations with a full text of about 6000 Dissertations, has been created by Nehru Library, Ch. Charan Singh Haryana Agricultural University, Hisar with financial support from Indian Council of Agricultural Research, New Delhi under its National Agricultural

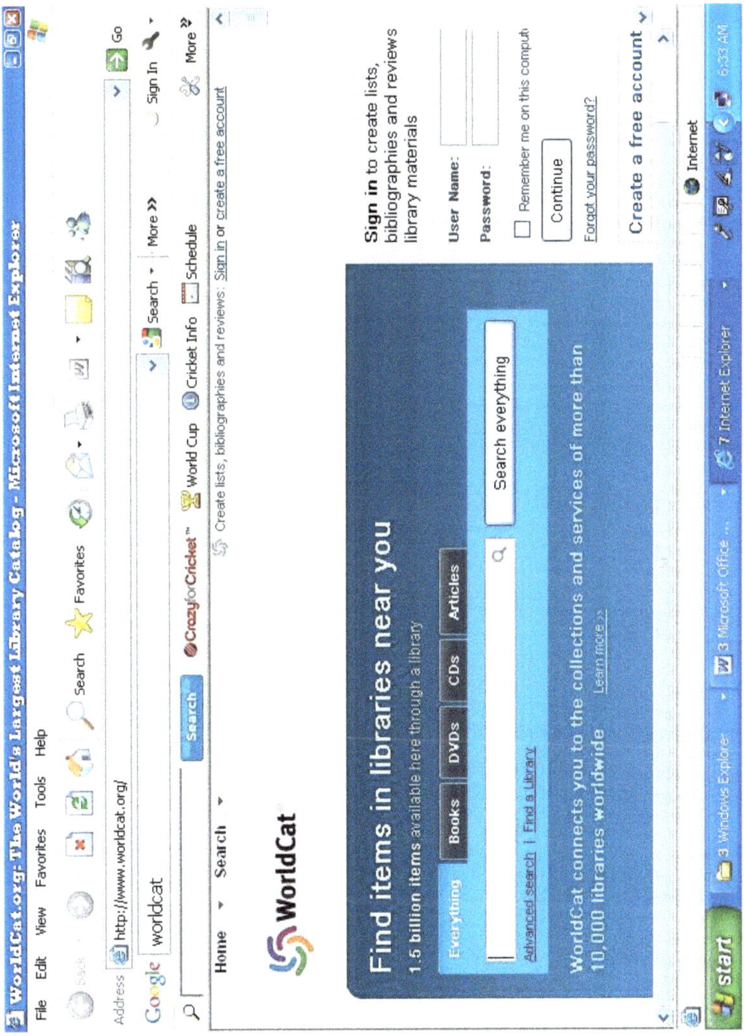
WorldCat.org: The World's Largest Library Catalog - Microsoft Internet Explorer
File Edit View Favorites Tools Help
Back
Search
Favorites
Address http://www.worldcat.org/
Go
worldcat
Search
More »
Sign In
CrazyforCricket
World Cup
Cricket Info
Schedule
More
Home
Search
Create lists, bibliographies and reviews: Sign in or create a free account
WorldCat
Find items in libraries near you
1.5 billion items available here through a library
Everything
Books
DVDs
CDs
Articles
Search everything
Advanced search | Find a Library
WorldCat connects you to the collections and services of more than 10,000 libraries worldwide
Learn more »
Sign in to create lists, bibliographies and reviews library materials
User Name:
Password:
Remember me on this comput
Continue
Forgot your password?
Create a free account
Internet
start
3 Windows Explorer
3 Microsoft Office ...
7 Internet Explorer
6:33 AM

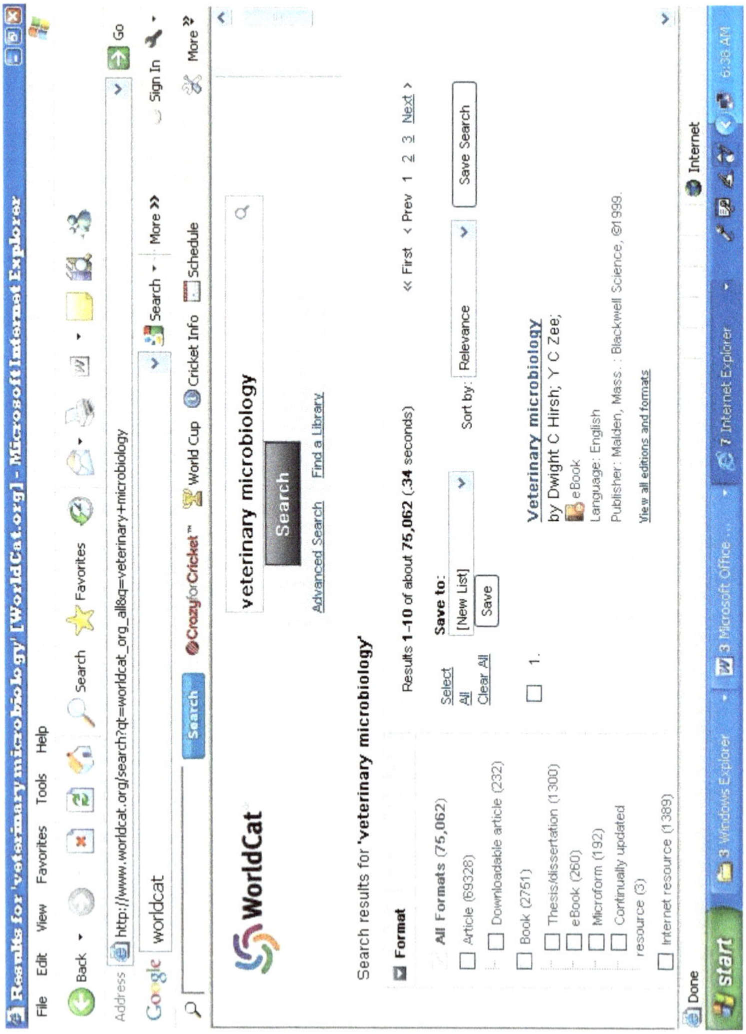
Results for 'veterinary microbiology' [WorldCat.org] - Microsoft Internet Explorer
File Edit View Favorites Tools Help
Back Search Favorites
Address http://www.worldcat.org/search?qt=worldcat_org_all&q=veterinary+microbiology
Go
worldcat
Search More
Sign In
Search
CrazyforCricket
World Cup
Cricket Info
Schedule
More
WorldCat
veterinary microbiology
Search
Advanced Search
Find a Library
Search results for 'veterinary microbiology'
Format
All Formats (75,062)
Article (69328)
Downloadable article (232)
Book (2751)
Thesis/dissertation (1300)
eBook (260)
Microform (192)
Continually updated resource (3)
Internet resource (1389)
Results 1-10 of about 75,062 (.34 seconds)
« First ‹ Prev 1 2 3 Next ›
Select All
Clear All
Save to:
[New List]
Save
Sort by:
Relevance
Save Search
1.
Veterinary microbiology
by Dwight C Hirsh; Y C Zee;
eBook
Language: English
Publisher: Malden, Mass. : Blackwell Science, ©1999.
View all editions and formats
Done
Internet
start
3 Windows Explorer
3 Microsoft Office ...
7 Internet Explorer
6:38 AM

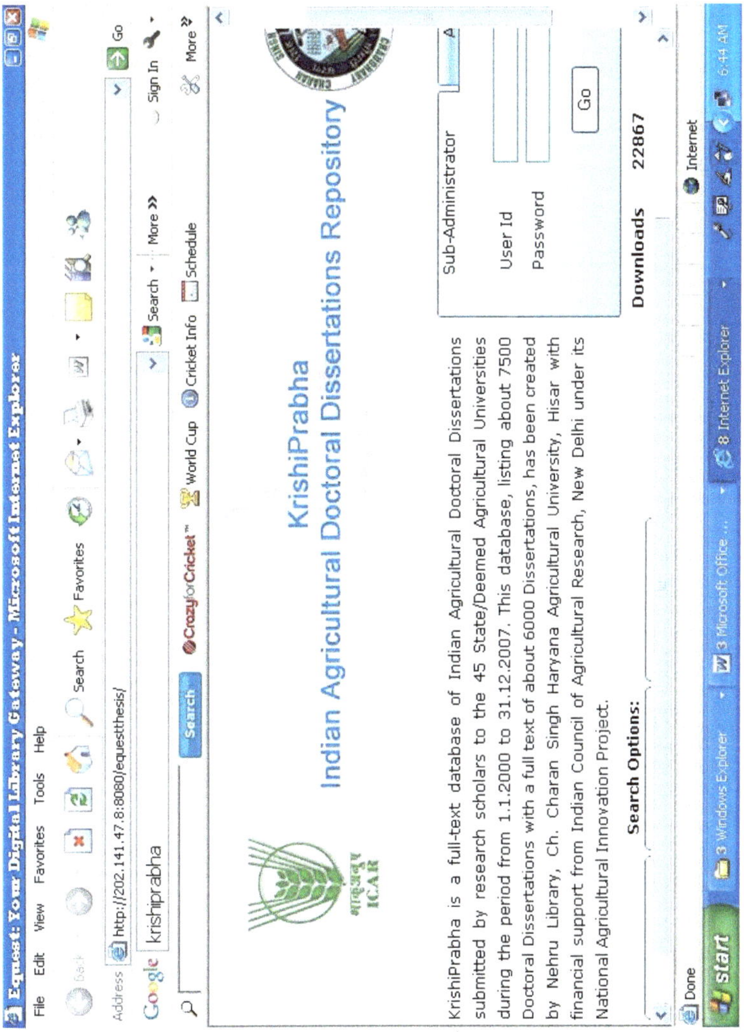

Equest: Your Digital Library Gateway - Microsoft Internet Explorer
File Edit View Favorites Tools Help
Search Favorites
Address http://202.141.47.8:8080/equestthesis/
Go
Google krishiprabha
Search More »
Sign In
CrazyforCricket World Cup Cricket Info Schedule
More
ICAR
KrishiPrabha
Indian Agricultural Doctoral Dissertations Repository
Sub-Administrator
User Id
Password
Go
KrishiPrabha is a full-text database of Indian Agricultural Doctoral Dissertations submitted by research scholars to the 45 State/Deemed Agricultural Universities during the period from 1.1.2000 to 31.12.2007. This database, listing about 7500 Doctoral Dissertations with a full text of about 6000 Dissertations, has been created by Nehru Library, Ch. Charan Singh Haryana Agricultural University, Hisar with financial support from Indian Council of Agricultural Research, New Delhi under its National Agricultural Innovation Project.
Search Options:
Downloads 22867
Done
Internet
start
3 Windows Explorer
3 Microsoft Office ...
8 Internet Explorer
6:44 AM

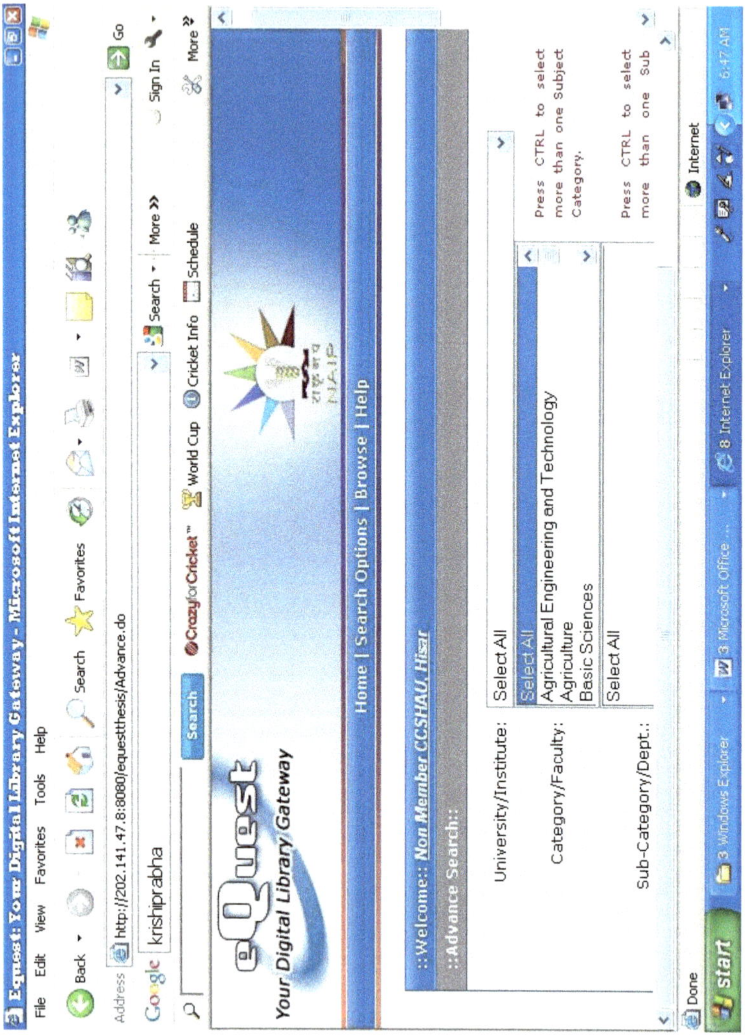
Equest: Your Digital Library Gateway - Microsoft Internet Explorer
File Edit View Favorites Tools Help
Back
Search
Favorites
Address
http://202.141.47.8:8080/equestthesis/Advance.do
Go
krishiprabha
Search
More »
Sign In
CrazyforCricket™
World Cup
Cricket Info
Schedule
More
eQuest
Your Digital Library Gateway
NAIP
Home | Search Options | Browse | Help
::Welcome:: Non Member CCSHAU, Hisar
::Advance Search::
University/Institute:
Select All
Category/Faculty:
Select All
Agricultural Engineering and Technology
Agriculture
Basic Sciences
Press CTRL to select more than one Subject Category.
Sub-Category/Dept.:
Select All
Press CTRL to select more than one Sub
Done
Internet
start
3 Windows Explorer
3 Microsoft Office ...
8 Internet Explorer
6:47 AM

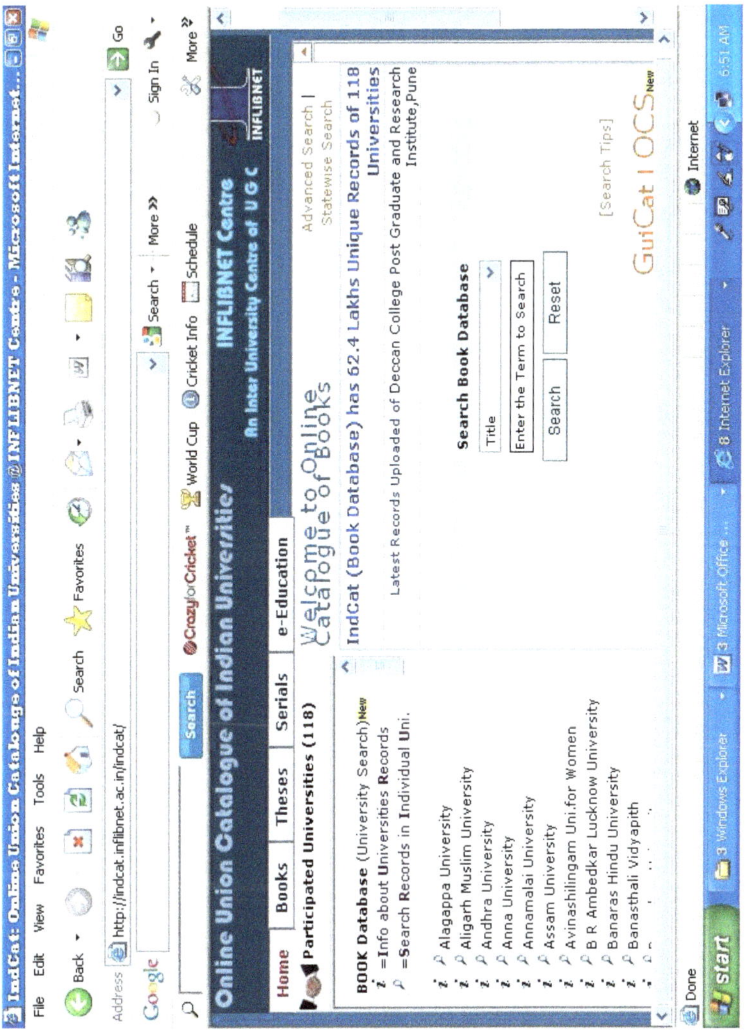
IndCat: Online Union Catalogue of Indian Universities @ INFLIBNET Centre - Microsoft Internet...
File Edit View Favorites Tools Help
http://indcat.inflibnet.ac.in/indcat/
Online Union Catalogue of Indian Universities
INFLIBNET Centre
An Inter University Centre of U G C
Home
Books
Theses
Serials
e-Education
Participated Universities (118)
Welcome to Online Catalogue of Books
Advanced Search | Statewise Search
IndCat (Book Database) has 62.4 Lakhs Unique Records of 118 Universities
Latest Records Uploaded of Deccan College Post Graduate and Research Institute,Pune
BOOK Database (University Search) New
=Info about Universities Records
=Search Records in Individual Uni.
Alagappa University
Aligarh Muslim University
Andhra University
Anna University
Annamalai University
Assam University
Avinashilingam Uni.for Women
B R Ambedkar Lucknow University
Banaras Hindu University
Banasthali Vidyapith
Search Book Database
Title
Enter the Term to Search
Search
Reset
[Search Tips]
GuiCat I OCS New
Done
Internet
start
6:51 AM

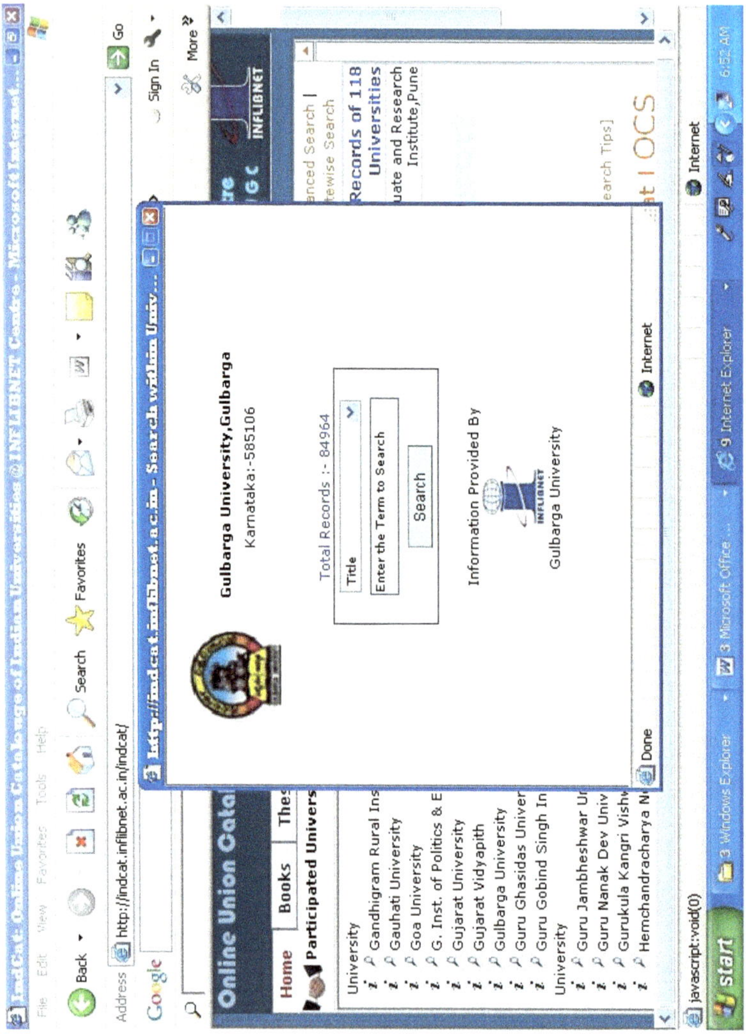

Address http://indcat.inflibnet.ac.in/indcat/
Online Union Catalogue
Home
Books
Participated Universities
Gandhigram Rural Institute
Gauhati University
Goa University
G. Inst. of Politics & E
Gujarat University
Gujarat Vidyapith
Gulbarga University
Guru Ghasidas University
Guru Gobind Singh In
Guru Jambheshwar Ur
Guru Nanak Dev Univ
Gurukula Kangri Vishw
Hemchandracharya N
Gulbarga University,Gulbarga
Karnataka:-585106
Total Records :- 84964
Title
Enter the Term to Search
Search
Information Provided By
INFLIBNET
Gulbarga University
Done
Internet
Records of 118 Universities
INFLIBNET
javascript:void(0)
start

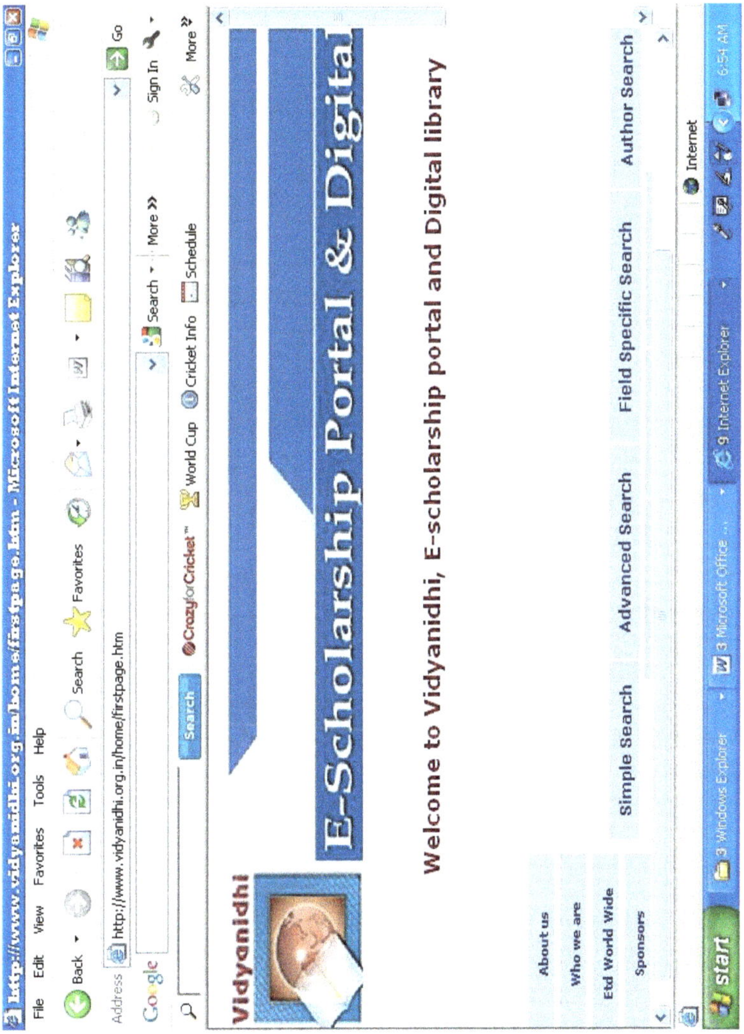
http://www.vidyanidhi.org.in/home/firstpage.htm - Microsoft Internet Explorer
File Edit View Favorites Tools Help
Address http://www.vidyanidhi.org.in/home/firstpage.htm
Vidyanidhi
E-Scholarship Portal & Digital
Welcome to Vidyanidhi, E-scholarship portal and Digital library
About us
Who we are
Etd World Wide
Sponsors
Simple Search
Advanced Search
Field Specific Search
Author Search
Internet
start

Innovation Project. This database makes provision to search by keywords, Category/Faculty, Sub-Category/Department, Author, Guide etc.

6.2.4 Union Catalogue of Indian Universities (http://indcat.inflibnet.ac.in/indcat/)

IndCat is an online Union Catalogue of Indian Universities provides Catalogues of books, theses and journals available in major university libraries in India. The union database contains bibliographic description, location and holdings information for books, journals and theses in all subject areas available in more than 123 university libraries across the country. A Web-based interface is designed to provide easy access to the merged catalogues. The IndCat is a major source of bibliographic information that can be used for inter-library loan, collections development as well as for copy cataloguing and retro-conversion of bibliographic records. The IndCat consists three components available in open access to users and librarians *i.e.* Books, Theses and serials subscribed in Indian universities.

6.2.5 Vidyanidhi - Digital Library and E-Scholarship Portal (http://www.vidyanidhi.org.in/)

Vidyanidhi refers to 'Treasure of Knowledge' in Sanskrit language and it is a India's premier Digital library initiative to facilitate the creation, archiving and accessing of doctoral theses. Vidyanidhi is an information infrastructure, a digital library, a portal of resources, tools and facilities for doctoral research in India. Vidyanidhi is envisioned to evolve as a national repository and a consortium for e-theses through participation and partnership with universities, academic institutions and other stake holders and it enhances access to Indian theses and enlarges the reach and audience for Indian doctoral research works.

References and Further Reading

De Gannaro, R (1977). Escalating Journal Prices: Time to Fight Back. *American Libraries*, 8: 69 – 74.

King, D.W. *et al.* (1976). Statistical Indicators of Scientific and Technical Communication (1960 – 1980). Vol.2. Rockville : King Research Inc., Centre for Quantitative Sciences.

King, D. W. and Tenopir, Carol (1998). Economic Cost Models of Scientific Scholarly Journals, - University of Tennessee School of Information Sciences Center for Information Studies - Paper presented to the ICSU Press Workshop, Keble College, Oxford, UK, 31 March to 2 April 1998.

Narin, F and Carpenter, M.P. (1974). National Publication and Citation Comparisons. New Jersey: Computer Horizons.

Price D. J. Solla (1961). Science since Babylon, New Haven: Yale U. Press.

Chapter 7

Internet E-Resources and Web Based Services

7.1 Origin of Internet

The history of the Internet starts in the 1950s and 1960s with the development of computers. This began with point-to-point communication between mainframe computers and terminals, expanded to point-to-point connections between computers and then early research into packet switching. In the 1950s and early 1960s, before the widespread inter-networking that led to the Internet, most communication networks were limited in that they only allowed communications between the stations on the network. The Internet had its developmental roots in the U.S. Military during the 1960s. A pioneering long-haul network funded by what's now-called DARPA (formerly known as ARPA). It was the foundation on which the Internet was built. The Advanced Research Projects Agency (ARPA) was funded by the Department of Defense and was a Cold War military project to test the possibility of creating a disaster-proof nationwide computer system. It was designed for purposes of military communication in United States devastated by a Soviet nuclear attack. The goal was to develop a peer-to-peer computer system - a radical departure from the conventional mainframe hierarchical system.

The Internet is actually a by-product of the Cold War. In the 1960s, the US Department of Defense (DoD) created ARPANET. ARPANET began as an experiment in reliable decentralized networking, linking the DoD with military contractors and universities funded to conduct military research. In the 1970s, additional North American Universities and research bodies joined the fray. In 1973, the first European Organizations were connected. It was also in the 1970s that Bell Labs UNIX began to rise to prominence as a solution for networked computing. Eventually, a second network, called MILNET, took over military traffic, while European (EUNET) and Japanese UNIX networks became established. In Europe, the United Kingdom set up JANET (Joint Academic Network). In 1986, the US National Science Foundation set up NSFNET, which linked five US university supercomputer Centres, a major milestone in the development of the Internet. Late in the 1980s, several US and foreign networks were becoming inter-connected, thus forming what is now known as the Internet.

The US Defense Advanced Research Projects Agency (DARPA) in 1973 initiated a research program to investigate techniques and technologies for interlinking packet networks with an objective to develop communication protocols for effective communication across multiple and linked packet networks.

During the due course of the development of Internet technology, the Internet system began to include support for other protocols into its basic networking structure. The system of protocols which was developed over the course of this research effort became known as the TCP/IP Protocol Suite, after the two initial protocols developed: Transmission Control Protocol (TCP) and Internet Protocol (IP). During 1980s, more than 100 protocols have emerged and in 1990s, an emphasis on the need of multi-protocol networking was placed. This resulted in development of Open System Inter-connection protocols (OSI) in 1991. The development of hypertext based technology called World Wide Web (WWW) provided means of displaying text, graphics, and animations, and easy search and navigation tools that triggered Internet's explosive worldwide growth.

7.2 Concept of Internet

Internet is a brand-new world with its own language. It is a computer network of networks. It is a vast information superhighway that facilitates communication between computer users both nationally and internationally. It enables computers of all kinds to share services and communicate directly as if they are part of a giant global computing machine.

With the arrival of Information Technology especially Internet technology in a significant way in India, Information, services and products are undergoing rapid changes in all sectors including the services being provided by the various government agencies to citizens.

India has been connected to the Internet since 1989. Currently, it is estimated that there are about 100 million Internet users in this

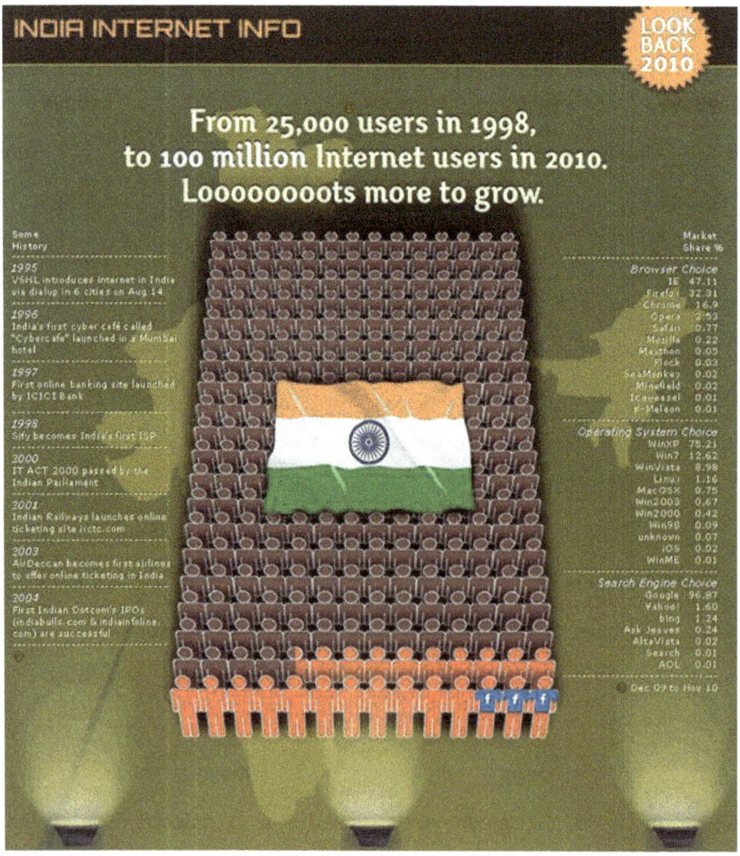
INDIA INTERNET INFO
LOOK BACK 2010
From 25,000 users in 1998,
to 100 million Internet users in 2010.
Looooooots more to grow.
Some History
1995
VSNL introduces Internet in India via dialup in 6 cities on Aug 14
1996
India's first cyber café called "Cybercafe" launched in a Mumbai hotel
1997
First online banking site launched by ICICI Bank
1998
Sify becomes India's first ISP
2000
IT ACT 2000 passed by the Indian Parliament
2001
Indian Railways launches online ticketing site irctc.com
2003
AirDeccan becomes first airlines to offer online ticketing in India
2004
First Indian Dotcom's IPOs (indiabulls.com & indiainfoline.com) are successful
Market Share %
Browser Choice
IE 47.11
Firefox 32.31
Chrome 16.9
Opera 2.53
Safari 0.77
Mozilla 0.22
Maxthon 0.05
Flock 0.03
SeaMonkey 0.02
Minefield 0.02
Iceweasel 0.01
K-Meleon 0.01
Operating System Choice
WinXP 75.21
Win7 12.62
WinVista 8.98
Linux 1.16
MacOSX 0.75
Win2003 0.67
Win2000 0.42
Win98 0.09
unknown 0.07
iOS 0.02
WinME 0.01
Search Engine Choice
Google 96.87
Yahoo! 1.60
bing 1.24
Ask Jeeves 0.24
AltaVista 0.02
Search 0.01
AOL 0.01
Dec 09 to Nov 10

Source: http://eyedealab.com/blog/article/india-internet-information-infographics/

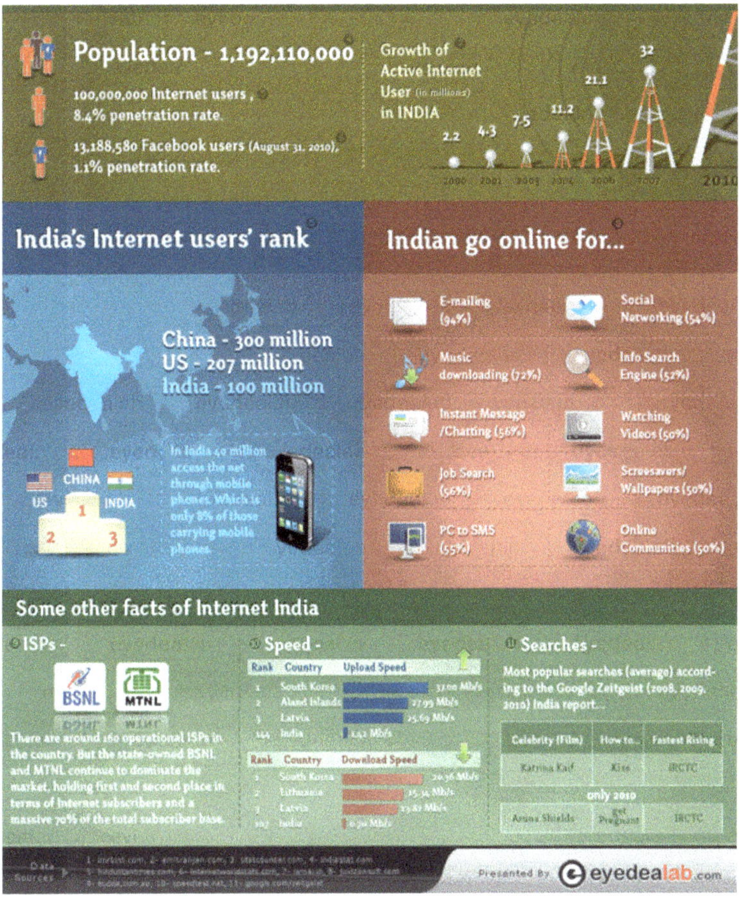

Source: http://eyedealab.com/blog/article/india-internet-information-infographics/

country. Access to the Internet is provided by four government organizations - Education and Research Network (ERNET), which provides service to the academic and research segments of society, National Informatics Centre (NIC) which serves government agencies, Software Technology Parks of India (STPI) which acts as a developer for software development companies, and Videsh Sanchar Nigam Limited (VSNL), which is the government's international telecommunications service provider. VSNL also provides the only Internet Connection available for the general public called Gateway

Internet Access Service (GIAS) and MTNL, Mumbai. Because the government owns/operates the entire ISP (Internet Service Provider) in India, government policy is the main constraint on Internet development. The Internet flourishes in an open competitive environment. The dominance/interference of a government in this industry is a negative factor.

7.3 Internet Web Browsers

The popular web browsers for Internet are listed below.

Logo	*Web Browser*
	Internet Explorer
	Firefox (also called Mozilla Firefox)
	Chrome
	Safari
	Opera
	Netscape Navigator

Logo	*Web Browser*
	Camino
	SeaMonkey
	K-Meleon
	Galeon
	Konqueror
	Maxthon Browser
	Flock (web browser)
	Midori

Logo	*Web Browser*
	Uzbl
	RockMelt
	Voyager
	Dillo Web Browser
	Slim Browser
	KidRocket
	Epic

7.4 Internet Services

With the tremendous volume of primary literature appearing every year in all the disciplines, the users need ways to become aware of new critical items they should be reading. The information service that provides the assistance to the users by libraries using information technology automatically search on most recent entries in a database for the benefit of users is termed as info-tech based information services. The various Info-tech based information services are discussed below.

World Wide Web

WWW (World Wide Web) is an Internet standard for distributed hypertext, in which the documents can have links to other documents that can be anywhere on the Internet. For example, if a document mentions "Constitution," clicking on that word might bring up a copy of the Constitution. Clicking on the Second Amendment might bring up a discussion of that topic, which might include links to articles at a completely different site, and so on. WWW is a *revolutionary* technology. Programs for browsing World Wide Web such as CELLO and Mosaic are available for most platforms, including Windows, Mac, X-Windows, and many more. Mosaic and CELLO are very nice GUI (Graphical User Interface) programs, which allow you to point and click to navigate most of the common Internet. It needs an IP (Internet Protocol) network connection to use WWW directly from the machine. However, one can also use a character-based program called "lynx" from your UNIX shell account to view WWW resources. With lynx, no images are displayed, but most of the info gets across. (Images are nice, but can also slow down WWW access a lot). With lynx, the IP connection is your service provider's which is likely much faster connection than your IP connection at home.

For a graphical WWW interface on your Windows machine, various Windows TCP/IP packages exist, including solid shareware ones like Trumpet, and good supported commercial packages from NetManage, Frontier and others. Most IP packages support serial protocols for connecting directly to the Internet over a modem.

E-Mail Service

In most academic and research institutions, e-mail has already become a replacement or alternative to internal memoranda. The ability to easily set up and maintain Internet mailing lists can be applied in the intranet context to support group communication. Mailing list can be archived and the archive made available from the intranet's web server to allow a group memory to be developed. Mailing list archives are also more accurate than traditional meeting minutes and means that groups no longer need to dedicate someone to make notes of their decisions.

Effective communication has been the need of the hour to bridge the time gap, which has enabled to communicate between the users around the world. E-mail refers to transmission of information from one person to another person electronically to foster time saving device. It is this technology that has minimized the popularity of postal services in the country for communication. Through this technology, the information in MBPS containing text, images, video, audio can be sent as an attachment in a very short time to the destination.

Library has been extending the e-mail service to the users and it has been widely used by the library professionals for carrying out library inhouse activities and services especially for ordering, enquiring or canceling order for documents and communication with peer groups; obtaining for reprints etc and are moving towards paperless society as far as communication is concerned.

File Transfer Protocol (FTP)

It is the Internet file transfer protocol/program used to transfer files. Using FTP to get files to the Internet-connected machine from other Internet machines. FTP sites listed here support anonymous logins, meaning anyone can use them by giving "anonymous" for Name and e-mail address as Password.

Telnet

Telnet is a facility through which logging into a remote site is much like logging directly there. Telnet sites are reference either by site name or numeric IP address. This application allows the user to login into the remote host, run software and read data files residing on the remote host. In most of the implementations of Telnet, a valid login and password is required.

Discussion Forums

A discussion list is a listing of e-mail names and addresses that are grouped under a single name. Through e-mail, everyone in the discussion group gets a copy of the message. These are frequently found on intranets, where they offer a kind of collaborative work area. Ideas can be exchanged on a variety of topics. Discussion groups are often managed using a list server operated using the same software that runs many Internet mailing lists. A number of freely available software packages are widely used, notably LISTSERV etc.

Newsgroups

Usenet newsgroups are like conferences or forums on a Bulletin Board System. Generally, anyone can read and post messages to a newsgroup. There are elaborate newsgroup hierarchies, starting with sci, talk, comp, alt, rec, and so on. Newsgroup postings expire after a certain amount of time regardless of whether read them or not.

Virtual Reference Service

Library services are being delivered to the remote users. New techniques in delivering information in various formats including electronic documents as alternatives to paper based documents. These methods of delivery include e-mail messages, FTP, putting information on bulletin boards or home pages on the Internet. This will avoid errors of transcriptions, reduce time and cost involved provides flexibility of timings and overcome barriers of distance.

Virtual Reference Service provides professional reference service to users anywhere anytime, through an international, digital network of libraries. This service is a real-time reference service via the Internet by making use of valuable resources. These advantages are possible because of digital uniqueness of documents and technology. The unique nature of digital reference introduces a new realm of issues and challenges. The need for guidelines and standards becomes even more important as consortium-wide digital reference services continue to evolve. Further, the improved facility of distribution and scanning make it possible to extend benefits to materials that are in non- digital format. The web, as a research tool allows the librarians to produce and deliver the information in electronic format, thus enhancing the level and access to a larger audience.

Online Public Access Catalogue

The library is a service-oriented institution which facilitates the users with its rich information resources through catalogue. With the advancement of Information and Communication technology, applications of Computer technology with dedicated library software's has enabled the libraries to develop new service known as Online Public Access Catalogue (OPAC) to the users. This reflects the library holdings in machine-readable format providing various searching access points like author, title, call number, Keywords etc.

The development of information technology and library software's in different platforms has enabled the library and information centers to host their bibliographical records on the Internet termed as Web OPAC. The OPAC in the networked environment is confined to the users within a campus, whereas the Web-OPAC extends its identity to the world by putting its resources made available in the bibliographical format. The Internet supports a variety of on-line services, and a number of tools are available to enable people to make good use of these, including: telnet, FTP, Gopher, Veronica, Archie, Wide Area Information Servers (WAIS), and the World-Wide Web (WWW). Now the library holdings are not only confined to library premises, but it can be hosted on the Internet revealing the collections of the library to the world. This facilitates the users to search the availability of documents in the library irrespective of location either by author, title, subject etc.

Document Delivery Service

Document Delivery is a term used in libraries to refer to the process of acquiring a copy of an item, which the home library does not own and does not intend to buy in the original. Thus, it could mean Inter-library Loan, the process whereby copies of books are borrowed from resourceful library to other libraries or copies of articles are obtained from them. As electronic journals become widely available, the boundaries between secondary abstracting and indexing services and the primary journals are obscured. Under Document Delivery Service, a print copy of the article/document can be delivered to the user using preferably Information Technology gadgets. The best example today are JCCC@UGC Infonet, JCCC@INDEST and JCCC@CeRa.

Content Alert Service

Contents alert services are available for free on the Internet. For instance, Elsevier's Science Direct is an example of a service offered by a major publisher that includes alerting services for their journals.

The options include a search alert that lets you input author names, subject words, etc.; a volume/issue alert to discover when a new issue appears; and a citation alert that notifies you when an indicated article has been cited by someone in a newer article.

The American Chemical Society (ACS) Publications Division offers a similar service for its 30+ journals, ASAP Alerts and Table of Contents Alerts. ASAP stands for "As Soon As Publishable," so when one of the articles enters the database, you are notified immediately via e-mail that includes a link to the article. The American Chemical Society - Table of Contents Alerts is also an e-mail notification service, but it comes out only when the entire contents of a new issue are posted on the Web.

Access to Full Text E-journals/Databases

Electronic media has become a day of demand due to information explosion leading to various e-resources to support academics. The users demand to access information at their desktops that too in electronic environment. As a result majority of publishers have started publishing print journals into electronic journals.

The major full text resources available including abstracting databases based on UGC Infonet resources are:

- ☆ American Chemical Society (31 Journals)
  http://www.pubs.acs.org/
- ☆ Royal Society of Chemistry (23 Journals)
  http://www.rsc.org/
- ☆ American Physical Society (8 Journals)
  http://www.aps.org/
- ☆ Institute of Physics (36 Journals)
  http://www.iop.org/EJ
- ☆ American Institute of Physics (19 Journals)
  http://www.aip.org/
- ☆ Cambridge University Press (72 Journals)
  http://journals.cambridge.org/
- ☆ Project Muse (222 Journals)
  http://muse.jhu.edu/journals
- ☆ J-STOR (293 Journals)
  http://www.jstor.org/

- ☆ Kluwer Journals (650 Journals)
  http://www.kluweronline.com/
- ☆ Springer Journals (550 Journals)
  http://www.springerlink.com/
- ☆ Emerald (28 Journals)
  http://www.emeraldinsight.com
- ☆ Nature (1 Journals)
  http://www.nature.com/
- ☆ Science Online (1 Journals)
  http://www.scienceonline.org/
- ☆ Encyclopaedia Britannica
  http://search.eb.com/
- ☆ Elsevier Science (34 Journals)
  http://www.sciencedirect.com/

ABSTRACTING DATABASES

- ☆ Chemical Abstracts Service
  http://stnweb.cas.org/
- ☆ Biological Abstracts
  http://web5.silverplatter.com/webspirsstart.ws?customer=c180470
- ☆ Royal Society of Chemistry (6 Databases)
  http://www.rsc.org/
- ☆ Analytical Abstracts
  http://www.rsc.org/is/database/aahome.htm
- ☆ Catalysts and Catalyzed Reactions
  http://www.rsc.org/is/database/ccrpub.htm
- ☆ Chemical Hazards in Industry
  http://www.rsc.org/is/database/chihome.htm
- ☆ Laboratory Hazards Bulletin
  http://www.rsc.org/is/database/lhbhome.htm
- ☆ Methods in Organic Synthesis
  http://www.rsc.org/is/database/moshome.htm
- ☆ Natural Product Update
  http://www.rsc.org/is/database/npuhome.htm

E-PORTALS

- ☆ Ingenta - Gateway Portal
  http://www.ingenta.com/
- ☆ J-Gate Gateway Portal - Informatics India Ltd.
  http://www.j-gate.informindia.co.in/

JCCC@CeRA-ICAR www.cera.jccc.in/

Agricultural research, the backbone of agricultural growth in the country, demands timely dissemination of knowledge being generated and updated across the globe from time to time. With the advent of internet facilities and advancement of web technology, almost all reputed international journals are available on-line and can easily be accessed by researchers over the network. Since ICAR is having network connectivity across the institutes and state agricultural universities, select journals could be made available over the network for the use of scientific community. Keeping this broad objective in mind, the NAIP has established the Consortium for e-Resources in Agriculture (CeRA) at the Indian Agricultural Research Institute (IARI). The NAIP is to facilitate accelerated and sustainable transformation of Indian agriculture in support of poverty alleviation and income generation by collaborative development and application of agricultural innovation by the public research organizations in partnership with the farmer's groups, the private sector, the civil society organizations and other stakeholders.

CeRA provides online accessibility of all important journals related to agriculture and biotechnology to researchers and students of the Consortium Partners and timely access to world R and D information and caters to the improvement of the quality of scientific publications, and teaching and research guidance.

CeRA is consortium of e-journals being subscribed by NAIP, ICAR and access is provided to 123 libraries of Agriculture (NARS) for the years 2008-10 (3 years). Through this service the user can access the following three major on-line Portals and Bouquet of Journals from Publishers with full text of an article.

- ☆ **Springer link:** It is a platform of Springer and product of bouquet of e-journals on different Subjects published by Springer. Through this Bouquet, user can access the full text of around 1100+ journals since 1996.

- **Annual Reviews:** Annual Reviews are authoritative, analytic reviews in 34 focused disciplines within the Biomedical, Life, Physical, and Social Sciences etc.
- **CSIRO (Australia):** Australia's Commonwealth Scientific and Industrial Research Organization (CSIRO)
- **JCCC (J-Gate Custom Content for Consortia):** It is a Contents' database collected from journals being subscribed by all 123 Libraries individually for the year 2008 (not through Consortium) under NARS. This database is customized product of M/S Informatics, Bangalore and covers the contents of only periodicals of electronic version and also gives link to approximately 4000+ open access journals since year 2000.

AGRIS

The Agricultural Resources Information System (AgRIS) is the Central Sector Scheme for Strengthening/Promoting Agricultural Information System in the Department of Agriculture and Cooperation (DAC), Ministry of Agriculture, Government of India. agris.nic.in/agrisportaljuly08.doc

7.5 Internet Resources for Agricultural and Veterinary Databases

Veterinary professionals and researchers need information through web sources to accomplish for their research work and patient care. Unfortunately, the Web has a large number of documents that are irrelevant to their work, even those documents that are irrelevant to their work, even those documents that purport to be veterinary related. The Internet and its distributed, unorganized repositories, of information have compounded the problem of information retrieval. In addition to information overload, there is the vocabulary problem with respect to the retrieval of relevant information from systems. Often a veterinary information searcher is uncertain about his exact questions and unfamiliar with veterinary terminology. Veterinary search has several unique requirements that distinguish itself from traditional Web search. The lack – of diversity problem is aggravated by the nature of veterinary web pages. Hence , search results provided by existing medical Web search engines often contain much semantic redundancy, which cannot be easily handled by existing methods for identifying near-duplicate documents of result diversification. To find useful veterinary information, the searcher often has to go through a large number of Web pages laboriously.

Most of the web search engines allow the Searcher to use Boolean logic and truncation in search statements, typically, a search engine works by sending out a spider to fetch as many documents as possible, another program, called an indexer, then reads these documents and creates an index based on the words contained in each document. Each web search engine uses a proprietary algorithm to create its indices such that, ideally, only meaningful results are returned for each query.

Since the conceptualization of ICT, many of its websites are providing information, links and are acting as resource pages for the veterinary sciences. Currently available resources on the web about the veterinary sciences, which are of great research value to the teaching faculty and students in the field of Veterinary Sciences are given below.

Intute (www.intute.ac.uk)

Intute is a gateway to evaluated, quality Internet resources in animal health, aimed at students, researchers, academics and practitioners in animal health.

PubMed (www.ncbi.nlm.nih.gov)

Since July 1997 the National Library of Medicine based in the United States has provided free Internet access to Medline. Many sites now offer Medline access. The Library recommends the official Pubmed site.

Medline (MEDlars onLINE) is a bibliographic database covering the fields of medicine, nursing, dentistry, veterinary medicine, the health care system, and the preclinical sciences. Medline is a massive database of bibliographic citations (e.g., authors, title, and journal reference) and author abstracts from over 3,800 biomedical journals. Medline contains over 9 million records dating back to 1966 and has world-wide coverage, although the majority of citations are in English.

The bibliographic details can be printed off the screen. Ask the Library if you require the full text of the articles.

Animal Science (www.animalscience.com)

This new subscription site replaces the original site. It provides a searchable, comprehensive animal health and production abstract database with 25-year archive and linkage to full text primary journals in the Ingenta Journals system. Subject-focused community areas incorporating discussion forums and the facility for uploading documents. Visitors area with listserves, calendar, bookshop, useful links and much more.

Veterinary Faculty University of Montreal (www.medvet.umontreal.ca)

This database is produced by the University of Montreal and offers access to 125 veterinary journal titles and to 50 conference proceedings. It gives bibliographic details (title, author, journal title etc.) and abstracts to veterinary articles.

British Library Integrated Catalogue (http://catalogue.bl.uk)

This catalogue unites a number of previously separate sources to list over twelve million items in the British Library's outstanding collections.

NetVet (http://netvet.wustl.edu/vmla.htm)

NetVet has a comprehensive list of over one hundred e-mail discussion lists to keep abreast of latest developments in their respective field.

Search Engines

A **web search engine** is designed to search for information on the World Wide Web and FTP servers. The search results are generally presented in a list of results and are often called *hits*. The information may consist of web pages, images, information and other types of files. Some search engines also mine data available in databases or open directories. Unlike web directories, which are maintained by human editors, search engines operate algorithmically or are a mixture of algorithmic and human input.

In 1996, Netscape was looking to give a single search engine an exclusive deal to be the featured search engine on Netscape's web browser. There was so much interest that instead a deal was struck with Netscape by five of the major search engines, where for $5Million per year each search engine would be in a rotation on the Netscape search engine page. The five engines were Yahoo!, Magellan, Lycos, Infoseek, and Excite.

Search engines were also known as some of the brightest stars in the Internet investing frenzy that occurred in the late 1990s. Several companies entered the market spectacularly, receiving record gains during their initial public offerings. Some have taken down their public search engine, and are marketing enterprise-only editions, such as Northern Light. Many search engine companies were caught up in the dot-com bubble, a speculation-driven market boom that peaked in 1999 and ended in 2001.

Around 2000, Google's search engine rose to prominence. The company achieved better results for many searches with an innovation called PageRank. This iterative algorithm ranks web pages based on the number and PageRank of other web sites and pages that link there, on the premise that good or desirable pages are linked to more than others. Google also maintained a minimalist interface to its search engine. In contrast, many of its competitors embedded a search engine in a web portal.

By 2000, Yahoo! was providing search services based on Inktomi's search engine. Yahoo! acquired Inktomi in 2002, and Overture (which owned AlltheWeb and AltaVista) in 2003. Yahoo! switched to Google's search engine until 2004, when it launched its own search engine based on the combined technologies of its acquisitions.

Microsoft first launched MSN Search in the fall of 1998 using search results from Inktomi. In early 1999 the site began to display listings from Looksmart blended with results from Inktomi except for a short time in 1999 when results from AltaVista were used instead. In 2004, Microsoft began a transition to its own search technology, powered by its own web crawler (called msnbot).

Microsoft's rebranded search engine, Bing, was launched on June 1, 2009. On July 29, 2009, Yahoo! and Microsoft finalized a deal in which Yahoo! Search would be powered by Microsoft Bing technology.

Timeline (Full list)

Year	*Engine*	*Current status*
1993	W3Catalog	Active
	Aliweb	Active
	JumpStation	Active
1994	WebCrawler	Active
	Go.com	Active
	Lycos	Active
1995	AltaVista	Active
	Daum	Active
	Open Text Web Index	Active [2]
	Magellan	Active
	Excite	Active
	SAPO	Active
	Yahoo!	Active, Launched as a directory
1996	Dogpile	Active
	Inktomi	Active
	HotBot	Active
	Ask Jeeves	Active
1997	Northern Light	Active
	Yandex	Active
1998	Google	Active
	MSN Search	Active as Bing
1999	AlltheWeb	Active
	GenieKnows	Active
	Naver	Active
	Teoma	Active
	Vivisimo	Active
2000	Baidu	Active
	Exalead	Active
2002	Inktomi	Acquired by Yahoo!
2003	Info.com	Active
2004	Yahoo! Search	Active, Launched own web search (see Yahoo! Directory, 1995)
	A9.com	Closed
	Sogou	Active

Contd...

Table–*Contd...*

Year	*Engine*	*Current status*
2005	AOL Search	Active
	Ask.com	Active
	GoodSearch	Active
	SearchMe	Active
2006	wikiseek	Active
	Quaero	Active
	Ask.com	Active
	Live Search	Active as Bing, Launched as rebranded MSN Search
	ChaCha	Active
	Guruji.com	Active
2007	wikiseek	Closed
	Sproose	Closed
	Wikia Search	Closed
	Blackle.com	Active
2008	Powerset	Acquired by Microsoft
	Picollator	Closed
	Viewzi	Closed
	Boogami	Active
	LeapFish	Active
	Forestle	Active
	VADLO	Active
	Duck Duck Go	Active
2009	Bing	Active, Launched as rebranded Live Search
	Yebol	Active
	Mugurdy	Closed due to a lack of funding
	Goby	Active
2010	Yandex	Active, Launched global (English) search
	Cuil	Closed
	Blekko	Active
	Viewzi	Closed due to a lack of funding
	Yummly	Active
2011	Exalead	Acquired by Dassault Systèmes

Useful E-resources on Veterinary Sciences

Examples

- ☆ http://netvet.wustl.edu/vetmed.htm
- ☆ http://www.altvetmed.com
- ☆ http://www.animalscience.com
- ☆ http://www.bmn.com
- ☆ http://cahpwww.nbc.upenn.edu
- ☆ http://cattlepage.com
- ☆ http://www.msstate.edu.dept/poultry/disbact.html
- ☆ http://www.msstate.edu/dept/poultry/disviral.html
- ☆ http://www.msstate.edu/dept/poultry/disproto.html
- ☆ http://www.ultimateungulate.com
- ☆ http://vet.cabweb.org
- ☆ http://www.vet.net
- ☆ http://www.vet-software.com
- ☆ http://www.tulance.edu/-dmsander/garryfavweb.html
- ☆ http://www.ozemail.com.au/-academi
- ☆ http://www.ianr.unl.edu/pubs/animaldiseases
- ☆ http://www.aahc.com.au
- ☆ http://www.avama.org/care4pests/avmaanim.htm
- ☆ http://www.grandin.com/reference/handle.streess.html
- ☆ http://avma.org/care4pets
- ☆ http://www.ghrandin.com/reference/new.corral.html
- ☆ http://helios.bto.ed.c.uk/mbx/fgn/pnb/filbio.html
- ☆ http://hammock.ifas.ufl.edu/txt/fairs/49696
- ☆ http://www.airtime.co.uk/bse/welcome.htm
- ☆ http://inet.uni-c.dk/-iaotb/bse.htm
- ☆ http://www.vetmed.auburn.edu/-brockkv/bvdv
- ☆ http://www.admin.ch/bvet/BSE/Index.html
- ☆ http://res.ogr.ca/CDRN/main.htm
- ☆ http://acmepet.com./canine/genetic/index.html
- ☆ http://funnelweb.utcc.utk.edu/-ypd634/webtopic.html:

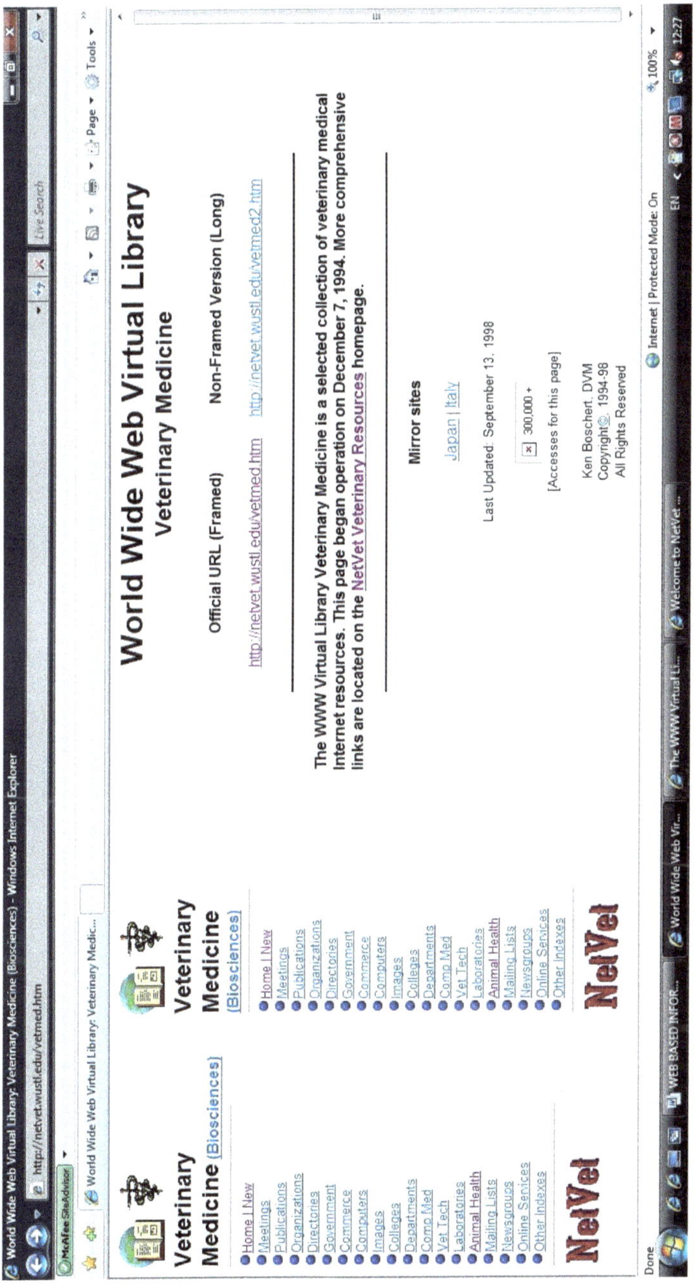

www virtual library: Veterinary Medicine

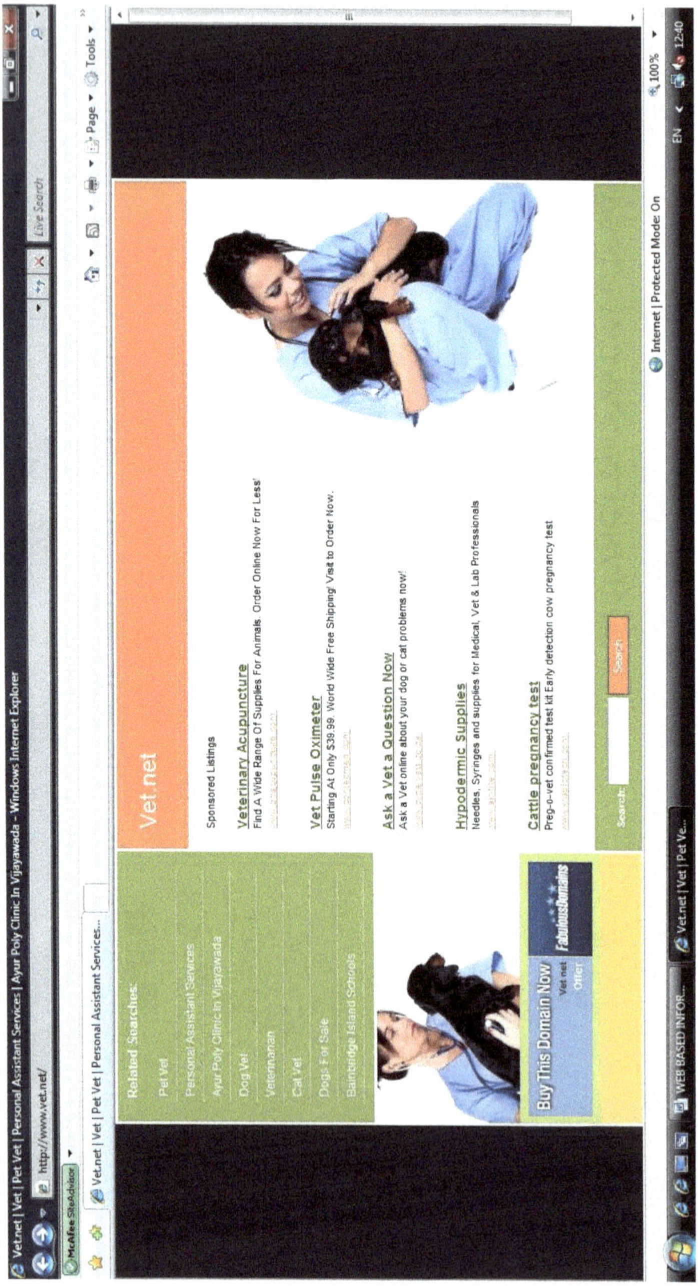

http://www.vet.net

- ☆ http://www.criver.com/techdocs/index.html
- ☆ http://www.aqualink.com/disease/sdisease.html
- ☆ http://freespace.virgin.net/larry.taylor/cavtpuk.htm
- ☆ http://www.ansci.cornell.edu/plants.html
- ☆ http://www-cyanosite.bio.purduce.edu
- ☆ http://mendel.berkelley.edu/dog.html
- ☆ http://www.grandin.com
- ☆ http://www.ecoli.cas.psu.edu
- ☆ http://www.avama.org/ezoo
- ☆ http://members.com/henryhbk/index.html
- ☆ http://www.Ishtm.ac.uk/mp/bcu/enta
- ☆ http://www.uky.edu/Agriculture/VetScience/Parasitology/home.htm
- ☆ http://www.cyberhorse.net.au/csl/tetanus.htm
- ☆ http://hammock.ifas.ufl.edu/txt/fairs/fairs/49680
- ☆ http://www.horseshoes.com
- ☆ http://ss.niah.affrc.go.jp/OIE/FMD/FMD.html
- ☆ http://www.lib.uiowa.edu/hardin/md/micro.html
- ☆ http://www.CyberArk.com/animal/holistic.html
- ☆ http://www.vetmed.ucdavis.edu/gdc/html
- ☆ http://www.ruu.nl/tropical.ticks
- ☆ http://agweb.clemson.edu/AgNews/Publications/ADVS/LL17.pdf
- ☆ www.vetmed.wisc.edu/pbs/johnes
- ☆ www.uel.ac.uk/pers/d.p.humber/hleish2.html
- ☆ www.vet.bg.yu/lepto
- ☆ http://www-sv.cict.fr/bacterio
- ☆ www.lymenet.org
- ☆ www.wam.umd.edu/-marky/mastitis.html
- ☆ www.segi.be/cemu/genetique
- ☆ www.naturalholistic.com:
- ☆ http://oncolink.upenn.edu/specialty/vet onc
- ☆ http://www.biosci.ohio-state.edu/-parasite/home.html

- ☆ www.life.sci.qut.edu.au/LIFESCI/darben/paraqut.html
- ☆ www.iah.bbsrc.ac.uk/virus/picornaviridae
- ☆ http://www.ianr.unl.edu/pubs/animaldisease/nf28.html
- ☆ www.rabbit.org/faq
- ☆ http://rotavirus.com
- ☆ http://numbat.murdoch.edu.au/spermatology/spermhp.html
- ☆ www.shoal.net.au/-rwylie/tikfaq.html
- ☆ http://www.parasitology.org
- ☆ http://cheval.vet.gla.ac.uk/vetscape
- ☆ http://vin.com/oncology/index.html
- ☆ http://life.anu.edu.au/viruses/welcome.html
- ☆ http://www.cvm.edu/wmc
- ☆ http://biodiversity.bio.uno.edu/-fungi
- ☆ http://medicine.bu.edu/dshapiro/zool.html
- ☆ http//www.vet.cornell.edu/consultont/consult.asp
- ☆ http//www.internets.com/sveterin.html
- ☆ http//www.nnlm.nih.gov/pnr/samplers/vetmed.html

Homepages of Organizations and Institutions

- ☆ http//www.cabi.org
- ☆ http//www.cgiar.org/ilri
- ☆ http//www.fao.org
- ☆ http://www.icar.org
- ☆ http://www.oie.int
- ☆ http//www.wehn.com
- ☆ http://www.nic.in/icar/cicfri.html
- ☆ http://cirg.up.nic.in
- ☆ http://www.nic.in/ciba
- ☆ http://gau.guj.nic.in

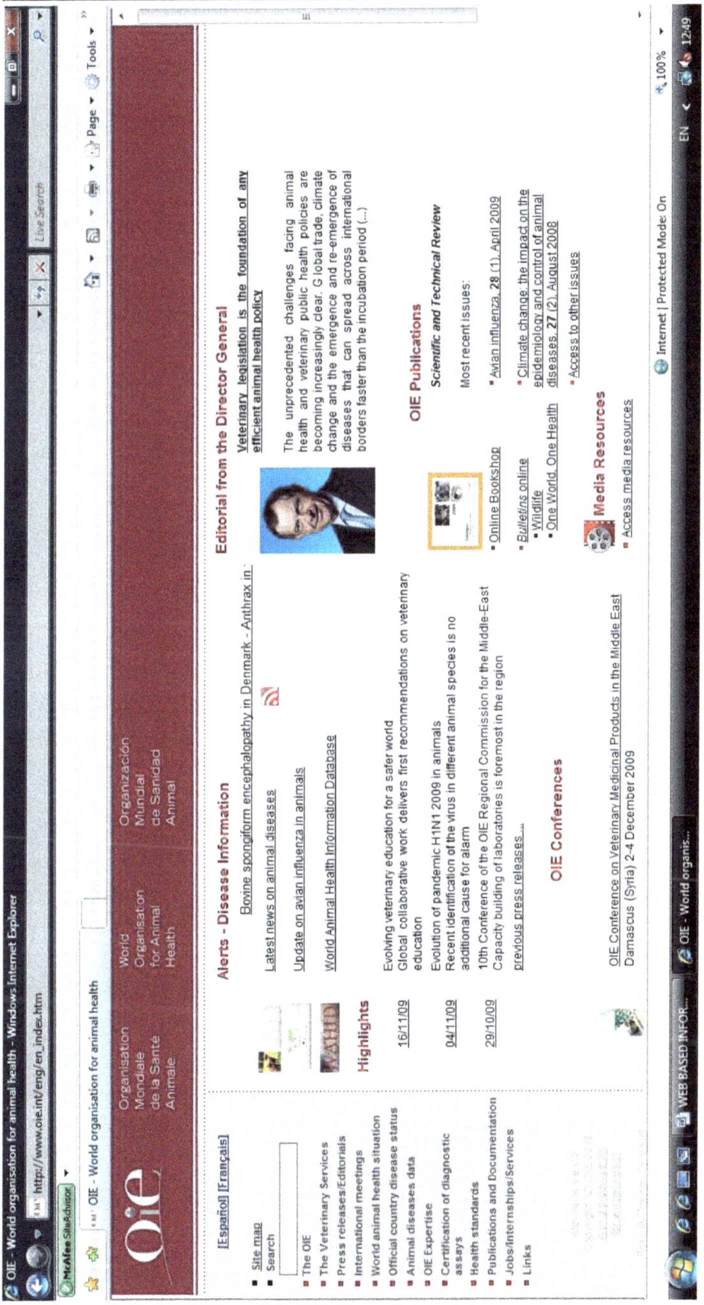

http://www.oie.int

Bibliographic Databases

It has already been mentioned earlier that many developing countries have their documentation centers which have created their own databases in different fields of agriculture. The advanced countries have brought their agricultural data in electronic, form, where as in India the agricultural information system is still in the formative stage. The Indian agricultural databases on tobacco (CTRI, Rajamundry), Diary (NDRI, Karnal) jute and sun hemp (JTRI, Kolkata), Plantation crops (CPCRI, Karsargod), Agricultural crops (IARI, New Delhi), dryland agricultural (CRIDA, Hyderabad), Potato (CPRI, Simla) etc., are still used in hard copy form. Happily CPRI (Simla) have created a machine readable database on potato in India comprising over 6000 references from 1901 to date. Here it will be appropriate to make a brief mention of the 'Bibliography of Indian Agriculture' (BIA) created by the Indian Agricultural Research institute Library, New Delhi, which is still handled and used manually.

Bibliography of Indian Agriculture (BIA)

BIA is also termed as Indian Agricultural Reference Media. It is a bibliographic database with author title references with citations on catalogue card form. BIA is being created since 1944 and today it contains about 1, 80,000 references. It covers Indian literature on plant sciences particularly on cereal crops, oilseeds, cotton, fruit and vegetables and medicinal plants.

Bibliographic Database with title Reference

Before the invention of CD-ROM technology, bibliographic, databases containing bibliographic references, citations etc were issued in printed form. However, most of them are still being published in print form parallel to CD-ROMs Almost of all these databases are computerized and are accessible electronically. To name a few are following.

- ✰ Bibliography of Agriculture (USDA, National Agricultural Library, Bethesda, Washington DC). It contains references only but no abstracts.
- ✰ Agrindex (FAO, Agris, Rome) (1975-1985). It contained references without abstracts.
- ✰ Science Citation Index (SCI) Institute for Scientific

information, Philadelphia, (USA). Science Citation Index is published in 6 series in annual comulations.

- Citation Index
- Permuterm subject Index
- Source Index
- Journal Citation Reports (JCR)
- Index of Scientific and Technical Proceedings
- Index to Scientific Reviews.
- Contain only citations (references cited in journals).

Bibliographic Databases with Abstracts

The most of the print version of agricultural databases contain abstracts- Substantive and informative in nature, which fulfill the information needs of users.

Some of the important bibliographic databases of this category are:

1. **CABI Databases:** CAB International London has built a computerized bibliographic database with abstracts to the tune of 3 million records since 1973. 1.6 lakhs records are added to in annually by scanning over 11,000 core agricultural journals along with books, monographs, conference proceedings, reports, bulletins, etc. It is the largest professionally developed database covering world wide issues in agriculture, forestry, dairy, animal and veterinary science, food and nutrition, etc. CABI database is published in 47 printed abstracting journals as well as on CD-ROMs. It is also accessible on Internet. (For details see CABI Abstracting Journals in chapter 10).
2. **Agris Database:** Agris (FAO, Rome) has built a bibliographic database since 1975. Up to 1985 it was purely a bibliographic reference database, but from 1986 it started indexing abstracts also. Presently, it covers only 21% abstracts indexing. Agris provides worldwide bibliographic coverage of agriculture, forestry, fishery, animal and veterinary science, food and nutrition, environment, etc. The Agris database is fully computerized and is accessible on Internet. It is also published on CD-

ROMs as well as in print form under title "Agrindex" (monthly service)

3. **AGRIKGOLA: Agriculture On-line Access (AGRICOLA)** is a bibliographic database created by the National Agricultural Library (USA) since 1970. Today, it is the most comprehensive source of bibliographic citations covering wide range of agricultural and allied subjects – Plant sciences, agriculture, animal sciences, aquaculture, veterinary science, forestry, nutrition, etc. It contains 3.3 million citations with abstracts to journal articles, monographs, theses, patents, reports, A-V materials, etc. 1,00,000 records are added annually. AGRICOLA is available online at NAL and accessible via the Internet as well on CD-ROMs and magnetic tapes since 1970. Its print version is 'Bibliography of Agriculture'.
4. **Biosis Database: Biosis** (Bioscience Information Service, Philadelphia) is the world's most comprehensive bibliographic database in the field of bio sciences, including life sciences, genetics, toxicology and zoological literature. Its Biosis Previews database on hard disk contains over 7 million bibliographic records with abstracts since 1985 and is available online as well as on CD-ROMs.
5. **Biotechnology Database:** Derwent Publications Ltd. Since 1982 have created a computerized database in the field of biotechnology scanning over 1200 world's leading scientific and technological journals. The online database is known as 'Biotechnology Abstracts' and its print version is also issued under title 'Biotechnology Abstracts'. It contains 140,000 Abstracts in the fields of biology biotechnology, chemicals, food and agriculture, genetics, health sciences, pharmaceuticals, plant genetics and breeding and wastes, etc.
6. **Chemical Abstracts Service (CAS):** It is the largest database in the world on chemical science and technology developed by the American Chemical Society (Ohio, USA). Since its beginning in 1907 Chemical Abstracts (CA) has published over 15 million abstracts for the CAS database (15 millionths abstract published on March 7, 1994). CAS

online database offers through STN Express a specially designed software package, a number of specific services like:

- ☆ Organic reaction information.
- ☆ Substances, hypothesized in chemical patents.
- ☆ Chemical formula, molecular structure of substances.
- ☆ Patents.
- ☆ Bibliographic references.

7. **Food and Human Nutrition Database:** FAO of the United Nations since 1975 have created bibliographic database which covers, food and agriculture, health sciences and nutrition, etc. It contains 3,11,000 records and adds 25,000 abstracts annually.
8. **Food Science and Technology Database (FSTA):** International Food information Service (IFIS) since 1969 has a world leading Food Science and Technology database which covers various aspects of food science, food products and food processing including biotechnology, economics, manufacturing, legislation and packaging for any commodity. Based on information from 2000 scientific journals in the line, FSTA database contains about 50,000 abstracts. Its hard disc information is accessible on Internet, in addition to CD-ROM and print copy of 'Food science and Technology Abstracts'.

There are many other computer based agricultural databases which are available on internet are:

- ☆ **Geobase (Elsevier Science Ltd)**: 1980 – to date 6, 00,000 records on hard disk cover geography, ecology, geology and mineralogy. Ground water and Soil Contamination Database (American Geological Institute) contains over 1, 45,000 records from 1975 to date. It covers chemistry, environment, soils, water science and technology. etc
- ☆ **Human Nutrition (CAB International)**: It contains 6,20,000 records on food and agricultural, health science and public health Life Sciences Collection (Cambridge Scientific Abstracts), Since 1982 it has held 17,47,000 bibliographic records on biochemistry, biotechnology, ecology,

entomology, genetics, immunology, health sciences, microbiology, toxicology, etc.

- **Plant Gene Database (CAB International)** covers over 4,50,000 abstracts on agriculture, biotechnology, genetics, genetics and plant breeding, food and nutrition, horticulture and forestry since 1973, and it available on internet and CD-ROM.
- **Toxline (Silver Platter).** National Library of Medicine USA supplies the majority of the information on Toxline with Silver Plater. Toxline on Silver Platter from 1966 to date offers over 2 million bibliographic references with abstracts. It covers information on chemicals, drugs, environment, hazardous wastes, health sciences, pollution and toxicology. It is available on Internet and CD-ROM.
- **Ulrich's International Periodicals Directory (R.R. Bowker Co USA):** A database of about 2,15,000 serial titles current and ceased, since, 1979, it available on Internet as well as on CD ROM.
- **Water Resources Abstracts (Cambridge Scientific Abstracts):** A bibliographic database contains over 2,50,000 records on Food and agriculture, environment, pollution, soil and water conservation, planning and government regulations, and it available on Internet as well as CD-ROM.
- **Wilson Biological and Agricultural Index (H.W.Wilson Company, USA):** A bibliographic database since 1983 to date holds over 5,50,000 references. It covers almost all aspects of agriculture, animal science and life sciences. It is accessible via Internet and also available on CD-ROM.

Reference and Further Reading

Bar-Ilan, J. (2004). The use of Web search engines in information science research. ARIST, 38, 231-288.

Bing Liu (2007). *Web Data Mining: Exploring Hyperlinks, Contents and Usage Data:* Springer.

Chhotey, Lal. (1998). Agricrultural Libraries and Information Systems. New Delhi:R.K.Teckno Science Agency.157 to 175p.

Chhotey, Lal and Bhatia, S. (1993). Adoption of Information Technology by Agricultural Libraries in India. *Annals of Library Science and Documentation*, 40(1): 4-11.

Javed Mostafa (February 2005). "Seeking Better Web Searches". *Scientific American Magazine*. http://www.sciam.com/article.cfm?articleID=0006304A-37F4-11E8-B7F483414B7F0000.

Levene, Mark (2005). *An Introduction to Search Engines and Web Navigation*: Pearson.

Malwad, N.M. *et al.* eds. (1996). Digital Libraries. New Delhi: New Age International Ltd. Publishers. Pp28-29.

Steve Lawrence; C. Lee Giles (1999). "Accessibility of information on the web". *Nature*, **400** (6740): 107.

Ralston, Anthony and Reilly, Edvin D. (1993). Encyclopaedia of Computer Science, 3rd London: Chapman and Hall.Pp413-14.

Ross, Nancy; Wolfram, Dietmar (2000). "End user searching on the Internet: An analysis of term pair topics submitted to the Excite search engine". *Journal of the American Society for Information Science*, **51**(10): 949–958.

For a more detailed history of early search engines, see Search Engine Birthdays (from Search Engine Watch), Chris Sherman, September 2003. Accessed on 4th June, 2011.

Index

www.ingramcontent.com/pod-product-compliance
Ingram Content Group UK Ltd.
Pitfield, Milton Keynes, MK11 3LW, UK
UKHW021623111026
15624UKWH00022B/7